SIMPLY
GLUTEN-FREE
& DAIRY-FREE

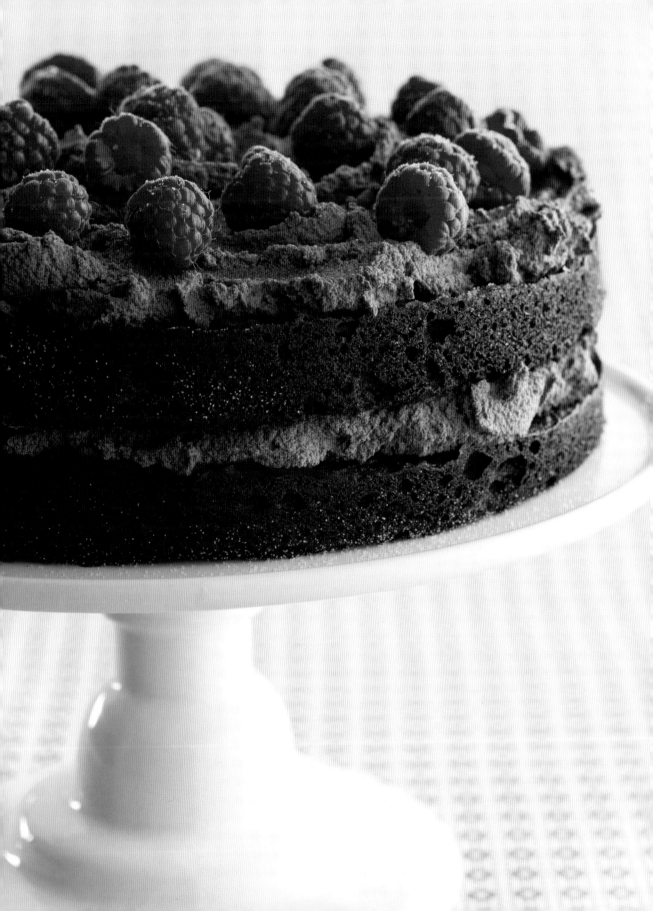

SIMPLY
GLUTEN-FREE
& DAIRY-FREE

BREAKFASTS • LUNCHES • TREATS • DINNERS • DESSERTS

GRACE CHEETHAM

dbp

DUNCAN BAIRD PUBLISHERS

LONDON

SIMPLY GLUTEN-FREE & DAIRY-FREE
Grace Cheetham

This paperback edition first published
in the USA and Canada in 2014 by
Duncan Baird Publishers, an imprint of
Watkins Publishing Limited, Sixth Floor,
75 Wells Street, London W1T 3QH

A member of Osprey Group

Osprey Publishing
PO Box 3985
New York, NY 10185-3985
Tel: (001) 212 753 4402
Email: info@ospreypublishing.com

Editor: Nicole Bator
Americanizer: Beverly LeBlanc
Managing Designer: Suzanne Tuhrim
Commissioned photography: William Lingwood,
except for the following by Toby Scott p.5 (bottom right),
59, 105, 141
Photographer's Assistant: Isobel Wield
Food Stylist: Bridget Sargeson
except for the following by Jayne Cross p.5 (bottom right),
59, 105, 141
Food Stylist's Assistants: Emily Jonzen and Jack Sargeson
Prop Stylist: Rachel Jukes

ISBN 978-1-84899-202-3

10 9 8 7 6 5 4 3 2 1

Typeset in Cambria
Color reproduction by Bright Arts, Malaysia
Printed in China

In loving memory of Pa, who was
the most wonderful father.

For information about custom editions, special sales,
premium and corporate purchases, please contact
Sterling Special Sales Department at 800-805-5489 or
specialsales@sterlingpub.com.

Publisher's note: While every care has been taken
in compiling the recipes for this book, Watkins Publishing
Limited, or any other persons who have been involved in
working on this publication, cannot accept responsibility for
any errors or omissions, inadvertent or not, that may be
found in the recipes or text, nor for any problems that may
arise as a result of preparing one of these recipes. If you are
pregnant or breastfeeding or have any special dietary
requirements or medical conditions, it is advisable to
consult a medical professional before following any of
the recipes contained in this book.

Notes on the recipes

Unless otherwise stated:
Use medium fruit and vegetables
Use fresh ingredients, including herbs and spices
1 tsp. = 5ml 1 tbsp. = 15ml 1 cup = 240ml

Author's acknowledgments

Huge thanks to everyone who has worked to produce such
a beautiful book, especially my brilliant editor, Nicole; my
Americanizer, Beverly; Suzanne for her design; William for
his photography; and Bridget for her food styling. Many
thanks also to Uzma for my author photo and to Duncan,
Bob and Roger, and the Sales teams. I couldn't have written
this book without the patience and support of my gorgeous
husband and daughter, Peter and Zoë, who light up my
life—and who put up with me writing and testing late at
night and at the weekends, and tasted everything for me.

Coeliac UK license number CUK-M-141

Watkins Publishing is supporting the Woodland Trust,
the UK's leading woodland conservation charity, by funding
tree-planting initiatives and woodland maintenance

www.dbp.co.uk

Symbols

GLUTEN–FREE
Contains no gluten-based grains or grain products, including wheat, barley, rye, oats, spelt, kamut, triticale, wheat bran, oat bran, and barley malt syrup.

DAIRY–FREE
Contains no milk, cheese, cream, yogurt, butter, or other dairy products from cows, goats, or sheep.

YEAST–FREE
Contains no ingredients with added yeast, including sourdough and yeast breads, all vinegars, wine, beer and other alcoholic beverages, yeast extract, Marmite, tamari soy sauce, and miso.

SOY–FREE
Contains no soy products, including soybeans, soy milk, soy yogurt, soy cream, soy cheese, tofu, tempeh, soy sauce, and soy-based margarines.

EGG–FREE
Contains no eggs or egg products.

NUT–FREE
Contains no nuts (almonds, Brazil nuts, cashew nuts, chestnuts, coconut, hazelnuts, macadamia nuts, peanuts, pecans, pine nuts, pistachio nuts, and walnuts) or nut oils.

SEED–FREE
Contains no seeds (flax seeds, hemp seeds, pumpkin seeds, sesame seeds, and sunflower seeds) or seed oils, including vegetable oil and seed-based margarines.

CITRUS–FREE
Contains no citrus fruit or zest, including oranges, grapefruit, lemons, limes, clementines, satsumas, and tangerines.

VEGETARIAN
Contains no meat, poultry, game, fish, shellfish, or animal by-products. May contain eggs or honey.

Contents

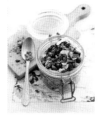
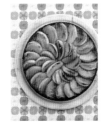
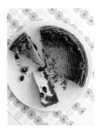
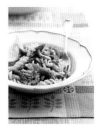
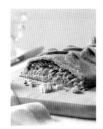

Introduction

For many people, food is a wonderful, enriching part of their life. But for those who have celiac disease or have allergies or intolerances, it can seem like a nightmare. When I was first diagnosed with intolerances, it felt as if the foods I was reacting to had become poisons to me, and that the whole culinary world had become a hostile place. It took time to learn to adapt my diet, but once I learned to make meals that I didn't react to, my relationship with food evolved. I accepted the changes and started to love food again.

I discovered ingredients that worked as alternatives to gluten and dairy, as well as ones that are naturally gluten-free and dairy-free. I worked out how to use different flours, grains, milks, cheeses, and yogurts, and found new ways to add flavor and taste.

As my life became busier, I learned how to fit my diet into my daily routine, making food I could easily take with me to work, when I was traveling, or before an evening out. Then when my daughter, Zoë, was born, I had to find ways to make recipes as quickly and simply as possible.

I've written this book in the hope that the recipes will inspire you to love food again, too. I've included dishes from all over the world, many of which use alternative ingredients to create gluten- and dairy-free versions of classics. There are recipes for all aspects of your daily life, including breakfasts you can eat on-the-run, lunches you can pack up and take with you, dinners you can cook for friends and family, and mouth-watering treats for any time of the day. But more importantly, I've based the book around simplicity. You'll find recipes that really are stress-free, with ingredients that work brilliantly, and techniques that will make purist cooks wince! Whip up the Brioche with Caramelized Peaches or Salmon en Croûte, for example, using a food processor, and you don't have to spend time kneading the dough or the pastry. Whiz cashew nuts in a blender to make cream for Chicken Tikka Masala or a Strawberry Pannacotta. Or use an electric mixer to make the crust for Herb and Olive Crusted Lamb or the batter for a Chocolate Birthday Cake.

For me, cooking is like alchemy—you take some ingredients and make a dish that can nurture you physically and emotionally. You can heap nutrients into your body—boosting your immune system, energy levels, and vitality, and helping your body to alleviate symptoms and start to heal itself. Then you can just sit back and enjoy the gorgeous tastes, textures, and aromas of the recipes you've created with each delicious bite.

Salt and Pepper Squid, page 64

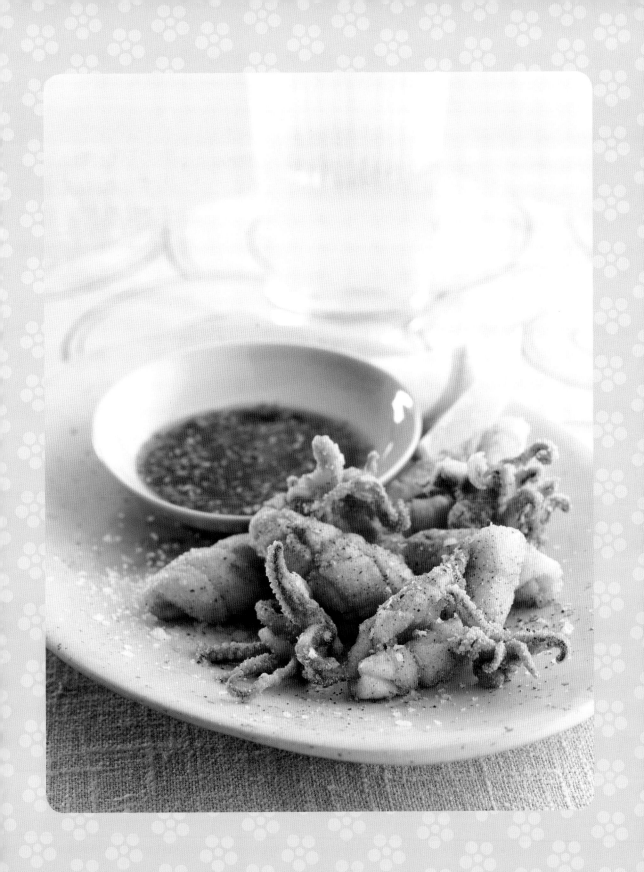

GETTING STARTED

It's well worth stocking up on lots of different ingredients so you have them on hand when you want to make something. Fill your cupboards with gluten-free pastas, noodles, polenta, and different types of rice. You can get fusilli, penne, spaghetti, and lasagne sheets made from corn and rice very easily. You'll also find wonderful varieties of rice noodles—thick and thin—as well as noodles made purely from buckwheat and glass noodles made from mung beans. Stock up, too, on dairy-free alternatives, such as margarine made from vegetable oils or soy, soy yogurts, soy cream cheese, and soy cheeses. They're fantastically useful, and most types last for a considerable time in your refrigerator.

For most of the baking recipes, I've used a mixture of rice, chickpea, and corn flours because they're easily available and they combine brilliantly in terms of flavor and consistency. I've also added potato flour to the breads to ensure they don't taste dry, like some gluten-free versions do. I've shown you how you can use other flours, too, so you can discover how to work with the different tastes and textures—and also benefit nutritionally. In the Buckwheat and Blueberry Pancakes, for example, I've used the nutty-tasting buckwheat flour, but combined it with sweet blueberries and honey so that the flavors sing. In the Chocolate Birthday Cake, I've added chestnut flour, which, unlike most gluten-free flours, has great binding properties—but its distinctive taste can sometimes overpower

other flavors. In this recipe, though, it goes perfectly with the rich, sweet chocolate and sharply sweet raspberries. And when I've used quinoa flour in the richly sweet Fruit Cake, I've masked the strong tastes of the quinoa with different dried fruits and ground almonds.

Quinoa is a wonderfully nutritious ingredient. I've used the flakes in the full-on fruity, nutty Apricot, Cranberry, and Goji Berry Granola (as opposed to buckwheat flakes in the Muesli) and the whole grain itself in the Roasted Vegetables and Quinoa, which shows how it works best with strong, bold flavors.

Amaranth is another wonderfood to add to your cupboard. The grain dates back to the time of the Aztecs and the Incas and can be used as an alternative to couscous, such as in the Pomegranate Amaranth. It's also a great bulking agent in the mixture for the Herb and Olive Crusted Lamb, giving the crust a really crunchy texture.

Cashew nuts make brilliant milk and cream. The textures are smooth and creamy and the nutty taste very subtle, making it hugely versatile. You'll find it in the dairy-free version of the fiery Chicken Tikka Masala, as well as in Strawberry Pannacotta and in the rich, thick chocolate frosting used in the Chocolate Birthday Cake.

Almonds are a classic gluten-free ingredient, used in many different cuisines around the world. Ground into a flour, they give sweet moistness in baking, as well as a nice light texture, such as in the Almond Cake. But they can also serve as a wonderful dairy-free alternative. As with cashew nuts, you can whiz almonds into a deliciously creamy milk or cream in your food processor or blender and make, for example, the irresistible almond cream to spread over the Almond Cake.

Coconut milk has finally lost its bad reputation and can stand tall as a high-quality dairy-free alternative. Although it does contain saturated fats, it's now acknowledged these fats are different from the ones in meat and, instead of being stored as fat in our bodies, they can provide a fantastic source of immune-boosting energy. Add in the high levels of vitamins that coconut milk contains, and you can tuck into the Chicken and Coconut Soup, for example, or the Shrimp and Butternut Squash Curry without any guilt!

It's also worth making sure you always have gluten-free tamari soy sauce in your cupboards, as well as a good gluten- and dairy-free bouillon powder, gluten-free baking powder, and lower-GI sweeteners, such as fruit sugar, xylitol, or agave syrup. Pick up some xanthan gum, too. It's brilliant at holding gluten-free baked goods together. Also stock up on cornstarch for thickening soups, stews, sauces, and fillings, and for creating a crispy coating, such as with the Salt and Pepper Squid.

As an alternative to cornstarch, I've also used kuzu, which is made from the root of a Japanese plant. Added to the Slow-Cooked Beef, for example, it creates a thick sauce. I've also used agar agar flakes instead of gelatin. Naturally processed from sea vegetables, these flakes are a staple in many Asian cuisines.

Sea vegetables themselves are brilliant. They add an exotic dimension to any dish, such as in the Arame and Cashew Nut Stir-Fry, and they supercharge the nutrient count of the dish. Add kombu to the Buckwheat Soba Noodles with Tofu, for example, and you create a fantastically nutritious stock.

I've used a couple of other unusual ingredients—umeboshi paste in the Duck with Plums and pomegranate molasses in the Cannellini Dip, the Lamb Burgers, and the Fig and Date Fruit Bars. Again, these are nutritious products that add delicious, distinctive depth of flavor to the recipes in which they're used.

As well as super healthy recipes, I've also put in lots of treats. You might want to keep sweet recipes to a minimum if you're watching your sugar consumption, but even if you only indulge every now and then, I wanted to make sure there would be lots of choice. Choose from breakfasts that will tempt you out of bed in the morning; cookies, cakes, and tarts to bring delight to your day; and desserts for true indulgence. Most of them contain significantly less sugar than conventional recipes and many have additional nutrients added. For example, the figs in the Chocolate and Fig Cookies provide calcium, potassium, and fiber. And the apples in the Apple Cake are rich in both soluble and insoluble fiber, which ease digestive complaints and help to detox your body.

In terms of equipment, try switching to PTFE-free nonstick pans that don't release

introduction

toxins, especially when frying at a high temperature. A food processor and blender, as well as a mini food processor or spice mill, are essential. Use them to spend minimal time and effort making the recipes—and to cheat whenever possible! I find it helps to keep this equipment on my kitchen counters. Without stopping to think, I can quickly chop tiny foods, like chilies, not to mention more time-consuming or tough things, such as nuts or lemongrass. And, oh, the complete and utter joy of mixing pastry dough in a food processor!

Baking with gluten-free flours can get messy! I get the best results when the dough has more liquid in it than a traditional dough, but this does mean the dough is very sticky. Gluten-free pastry can burn easily, too, so I also cover it with baking parchment. But don't worry—I've put step-by-step instructions in the recipes to show you how to handle the various doughs.

HELPING YOUR BODY TO HEAL

If you have celiac disease and have to avoid gluten, or suffer from other problems, such as eczema, asthma, migraines, nausea, vomiting, bloating, bowel problems, irritable bowel syndrome (IBS), chronic fatigue syndrome (CFS or ME), or depression, you might find certain foods aggravate your condition, and avoiding these foods will help enormously—that your symptoms will clear and you'll begin to feel much, much better. But your body's long-term reactions might well have had a hugely debilitating effect. Your adrenaline levels might have been high,

for example, causing your immune system to struggle, and you might not have been digesting food properly or assimilating the nutrients. So it is vital to replenish your body's store of vitamins, minerals, phytochemicals, and other nutrients so your body can start to heal itself.

Try to buy organic produce whenever you can, especially meat, fish, and eggs, and to eat pure, natural foods. Avoid additives or preservatives and check labels to see what's in the foods you buy—look for nitrate-free hams, for example, and unsulfured dried apricots.

Eat stacks of fresh fruit and vegetables, preferably local, seasonal versions that will have higher nutrient levels, as well as far superior flavor. Fill up with protein- and fiber-rich beans and legumes, including Puy lentils, chickpeas, fava beans, and cannellini beans. Add whole or ground nuts and seeds to your meals throughout the day, especially to juices and smoothies, muesli mixtures, salads, stir-frys, cookies, cakes, and desserts. Go for stable oils, such as olive, canola, or safflower, and add in essential fatty acids, particularly omega-3, through ingredients such as oily fish, walnuts, hemp seeds, and flaxseeds. Drink herbal teas and pure, life-giving water as often as you can.

ONWARD AND UPWARD

Above all, the recipes in this book are to be enjoyed. Dive into them with your family and friends and discover ingredients and dishes you love—whether for a quick snack, a super-healthy meal, or a truly magical feast.

Summer Pudding, page 159

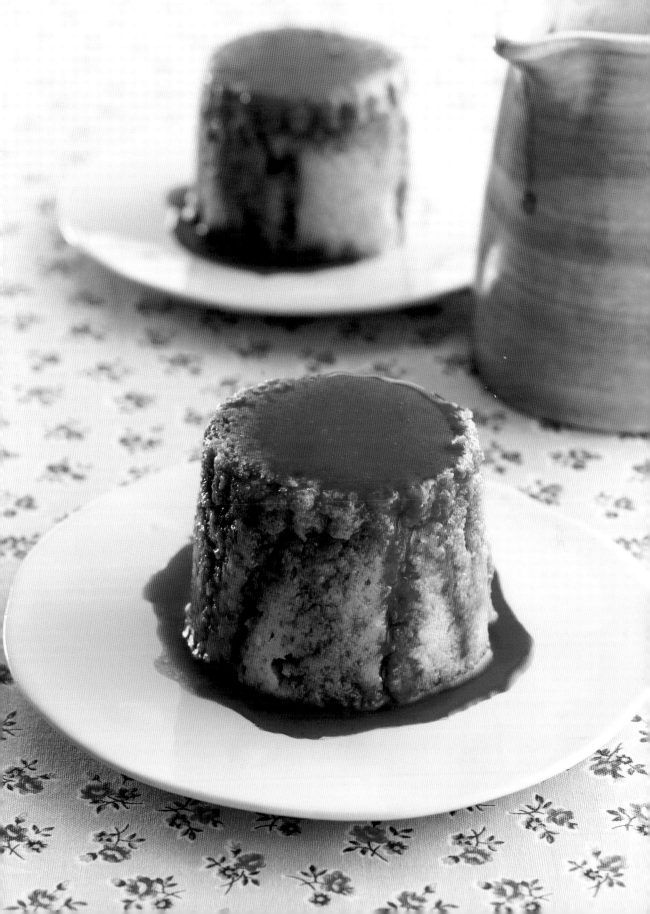

Basic Recipes

White Sauce

Makes **about 2⅔ cups**   Preparation time **5 minutes**   Cooking time **20 minutes**

3 tablespoons dairy-free margarine

heaped ¼ cup rice flour

1½ tablespoons chickpea flour

1½ tablespoons corn flour

2¼ to scant 3 cups Vegetable Stock
   (see page 21) or vegetable stock made with
   gluten- and dairy-free bouillon powder

sea salt and freshly ground black pepper

1   Melt the dairy-free margarine in a heavy-bottomed saucepan over low heat. Stir in the flours, then remove the pan from the heat and gradually add 1½ cups of the stock, stirring continuously. Return the pan to medium heat and bring to a boil, stirring continuously as it thickens. Gradually add another ¾ cup stock. If the sauce gets lumpy, beat with a whisk until smooth.

2   Turn the heat down to low and simmer very gently 10 minutes, stirring frequently to prevent the sauce from sticking to the pan.

3   Gradually stir in the remaining stock, if necessary, to make a smooth sauce that is thick, but still runny. Season lightly with salt and pepper.

Roasted Tomato and Pepper Sauce

Makes **about 5 cups**   Preparation time **5 minutes**   Cooking time **30 minutes**

3 red, orange, or yellow bell peppers, quartered
   and seeded

10 tomatoes, halved

1 large onion, peeled and quartered

3 tablespoons olive oil

2 garlic cloves

sea salt and freshly ground black pepper

1   Preheat the oven to 350°F. Put the peppers, tomatoes, and onion on two baking sheets and drizzle with the oil. Bake 10 minutes, then add the garlic and bake 20 minutes longer, or until soft and starting to brown.

2   Transfer to a blender and blend until smooth. Season lightly with salt and pepper.

Custard

Makes **about 2¼ cups** Preparation time **5 minutes** Cooking time **20 minutes**

2 cups plus 2 tablespoons soy milk

1 tablespoon cornstarch

5 extra-large egg yolks

½ cup fruit sugar or granulated sugar

1 teaspoon vanilla extract

1 Heat the soy milk in a heavy-bottomed saucepan over low heat until almost boiling. While the soy milk is warming, put the cornstarch and 1 tablespoon water in a large bowl and stir until smooth Add the egg yolks and sugar and whisk until the mixture thickens. Gradually add the hot milk and stir until well mixed.

2 Pour the mixture into a clean saucepan, add the vanilla extract, and cook over low heat, stirring frequently, 10 to 15 minutes until it forms a thick custard. Be careful not to overheat or the custard can curdle; if it does, beat with a whisk until smooth.

Cashew Nut Cream

Makes **about 2¾ cups** Preparation time **10 minutes, plus at least 12 hours soaking**

2⅓ cups cashew nuts

1 Put the nuts in a bowl, cover with cold water, and let soak at room temperature overnight, or at least 12 hours.

2 Drain and rinse the nuts thoroughly, then put them in a blender. Add 1 cup water plus 2 tablespoons water and blend 10 minutes, or until smooth.

White Bread

Makes **1 loaf (about 16 slices)**   Preparation time **15 minutes, plus 30 minutes rising**
Cooking time **50 minutes**

¾ cup potato flour

heaped ½ cup chickpea flour

scant ½ cup corn flour

scant 1 cup brown rice flour

1 teaspoon fine sea salt

1 teaspoon fruit sugar or granulated sugar

1 teaspoon gluten-free baking powder

1 teaspoon xanthan gum

1 tablespoon active dry yeast

2 tablespoons olive oil

dairy-free margarine, for greasing

1   Sift the flours, salt, sugar, gluten-free baking powder, xanthan gum, and yeast into a large
    mixing bowl and whisk to mix together. Add the olive oil and beat again, then add 1⅔ cups
    warm water and beat about 1 minute to aerate the dough. It will be sticky.

2   Cover the bowl with plastic wrap and let rise 30 minutes.

3   Preheat the oven to 400°F and lightly grease a 2-pound bread pan with dairy-free margarine.
    Spoon the dough into the pan and smooth the surface with the back of a metal spoon.

4   Bake 45 to 50 minutes until the bread is golden brown. Turn it out of the pan and tap the
    bottom. If it sounds hollow, it is done. If not, return the bread to the pan and bake 5 minutes
    longer, then test again to see whether it is done. Transfer to a wire rack to cool.

basic recipes

Rosemary Focaccia

Makes **1 loaf (about 10 pieces)**   Preparation time **15 minutes, plus 30 minutes rising**
Cooking time **50 minutes**

¾ cup potato flour

heaped ½ cup chickpea flour

scant ½ cup corn flour

scant 1 cup brown rice flour

1 teaspoon fine sea salt, plus extra for sprinkling

1 teaspoon xanthan gum

1 tablespoon active dry yeast

¼ cup olive oil, plus extra for greasing

1 handful of rosemary leaves, chopped

1 Sift the flours, salt, xanthan gum, and yeast into a large mixing bowl and whisk to mix together. Add 3 tablespoons of the olive oil and beat again, then add 1⅔ cups warm water and beat about 1 minute to aerate the dough. It will be sticky.

2 Cover the bowl with plastic wrap and let rise 30 minutes.

3 Preheat the oven to 400°F and lightly grease an 8-inch cake pan with a little oil. Spoon the dough into the pan and smooth the surface with the back of a metal spoon. Drizzle the remaining oil over the top, then sprinkle with the rosemary and salt.

4 Bake 45 to 50 minutes until the bread is golden brown. Turn out of the pan and tap the bottom. If it sounds hollow, it is done. If not, return the bread to the pan and bake 5 minutes longer, then test again to see whether it is done. Transfer to a wire rack to cool.

Flatbread

Makes **8**   Preparation time **25 minutes, plus 1 hour rising**   Cooking time **25 minutes**

2 teaspoons active dry yeast

1¼ cups brown rice flour

heaped 1½ cups chickpea flour

scant 1 cup potato flour

1 teaspoon fine sea salt

1½ tablespoons xanthan gum

2 tablespoons olive oil, plus extra for greasing

1   In a small mixing bowl, whisk together the yeast and 1¾ cups warm water and let stand about 5 minutes.

2   Sift the flours, salt, and xanthan gum into a large mixing bowl and whisk to mix together. Add the olive oil and beat again, then add the yeast mixture and beat about 1 minute to aerate the dough. It will be sticky.

3   Cover the bowl with plastic wrap and let rise 1 hour.

4   Preheat the oven to 400°F. Divide the dough into 8 equal portions and put 2 portions on a piece of baking parchment, leaving enough room to shape each one into a flatbread. Grease another piece of baking parchment and put it, oiled-side down, over the dough. Using your hands, flatten and shape both pieces of dough into flatbreads, each about ¼-inch thick. Remove the top layer of baking parchment. Transfer the flatbreads and bottom sheet of baking parchment to a baking sheet. Repeat with the remaining pieces of dough and arrange them on three additional baking sheets. Bake 20 to 25 minutes until lightly golden.

basic recipes

Corn Tortillas

Makes **8**   Preparation time **10 minutes, plus 15 minutes resting**   Cooking time **10 minutes**

1½ cups masa harina

1 teaspoon fine sea salt

1 Sift the masa harina and salt into a large mixing bowl and whisk to mix together. Add 1¼ cups plus 2 tablespoons warm water and beat about 1 minute to aerate the dough.

2 Cover the bowl with plastic wrap and let rise 15 minutes.

3 Divide the dough into 8 equal portions and shape them into balls. On a work surface, put 1 of the balls between two pieces of baking parchment and, using a rolling pin, roll it out into a thin circle, about 8 inches in diameter and ⅟₃₂ inch thick.

4 Heat a skillet or griddle pan over medium-high heat until hot. Cook a tortilla about 30 seconds until it has brown spots underneath, then turn it over and cook a few more seconds until it puffs up. Using a metal spatula, transfer the tortilla to a clean, slightly dampened dish towel and wrap it up to keep it warm and soft. Repeat with the remaining pieces of dough.

basic recipes

Light Pastry Dough

Makes **enough for 1 x 8-inch tart pan or 4 x 4-inch tartlet pans**   Preparation time **15 minutes, plus 30 minutes chilling**   Cooking time **15 minutes**

1 potato, peeled and cut into large chunks

⅔ cup brown rice flour, plus extra as needed

scant ½ cup chickpea flour

⅓ cup corn flour

½ teaspoon fine sea salt, plus extra to season

1 teaspoon xanthan gum

½ cup chilled dairy-free margarine, diced, plus extra for greasing

1 extra-large egg, beaten

1   Put the potato in a saucepan and cover with cold water. Bring to a boil over high heat, then turn the heat down to medium and simmer, covered, 15 minutes, or until tender. Drain, then mash the potato until smooth.

2   Sift the flours, salt, and xanthan gum into the bowl of a food processor. Add the dairy-free margarine and blend until the mixture resembles fine bread crumbs, then add the mashed potato and blend for a few seconds until mixed in. Add the egg and blend 20 to 30 seconds until the mixture comes away from the sides of the bowl and forms a sticky dough. There should be a little extra moisture at the bottom of the bowl. If it is too dry, gradually blend in 1 to 2 tablespoons chilled water. If it is too sticky, add a little rice flour.

3   Shape the dough into a ball, wrap it in plastic wrap, and chill in the refrigerator 30 minutes.

basic recipes

Piecrust Dough

Makes **enough for 1 x 8-inch tart pan or 4 x 4-inch tartlet pans** Preparation time **10 minutes, plus 30 minutes chilling**

⅔ cup brown rice flour, plus extra as needed

heaped ½ cup chickpea flour

scant ½ cup corn flour

½ teaspoon fine sea salt

1 teaspoon xanthan gum

½ cup chilled dairy-free margarine, diced

1 extra-large egg, beaten

1   Sift the flours, salt, and xanthan gum into the bowl of a food processor and blend well. Add the dairy-free margarine and blend until the mixture resembles fine bread crumbs. Add the egg and blend 20 to 30 seconds until the mixture comes together to form a sticky dough. There should be a little extra moisture at the bottom of the bowl. If it is too dry, gradually blend in 1 to 2 tablespoons chilled water. If too sticky, add a little rice flour.

2   Shape the dough into a ball, wrap it in plastic wrap, and chill in the refrigerator 30 minutes.

Sweet Piecrust Dough

Makes **enough for 1 x 8-inch tart pan or 4 x 4-inch tartlet pans** Preparation time **10 minutes, plus 30 minutes chilling**

heaped ½ cup brown rice flour, plus extra as needed

heaped ¾ cup chickpea flour

⅓ cup very finely ground blanched almonds

¼ cup fruit sugar or granulated sugar

1 teaspoon xanthan gum

5 tablespoons chilled dairy-free margarine, diced

1 extra-large egg, beaten

1   Sift the flours and xanthan gum into the bowl of a food processor. Add the almonds and sugar, and blend well. Add the dairy-free margarine and blend until the mixture resembles fine bread crumbs. Add the egg and blend 20 to 30 seconds until the mixture comes together to form a sticky dough. There should be a little extra moisture at the bottom of the bowl. If it is too dry, gradually 1 to 2 tablespoons chilled water. If too sticky, add a little rice flour.

2   Shape the pastry into a ball, wrap in plastic wrap, and chill in the refrigerator 30 minutes.

Chicken Stock

Makes **about 6 cups**   Preparation time **10 minutes**   Cooking time **3 hours**

1 large chicken carcass

1 onion, chopped

1 leek, white part only, chopped

1 celery stick, chopped

1 large carrot, chopped

6 parsley stems without leaves

1 bay leaf

6 black peppercorns

1   Break up the chicken carcass and put it in a large saucepan. Add all of the remaining ingredients and 2 quarts water. Bring almost to a boil, then turn the heat down to low and simmer, covered, 3 hours. Let cool a little, then strain into a container and let cool completely.

2   As soon as the stock is cold, remove and discard the layer of fat that will have settled on the surface. The stock will keep in the refrigerator up to 3 days or in the freezer up to 3 months.

Fish Stock

Makes **about 3 quarts**   Preparation time **10 minutes**   Cooking time **45 minutes**

4 pounds 8 ounces fish bones (preferably from
    white fish, such as cod, sole, or sea bass)

1 onion, chopped

1 leek, white part chopped

1 celery stick, chopped

1 large carrot, chopped

6 parsley stalks without leaves

1 bay leaf

6 black peppercorns

1   Wash the fish bones thoroughly and break them up into a large saucepan. Add all of the remaining ingredients and 3 quarts water. Bring almost to a boil, then turn the heat down to low and simmer, covered, 40 minutes.

2   Let cool a little, then strain into a container and let cool completely. The stock will keep in the refrigerator up to 2 days or in the freezer up to 3 months.

Vegetable Stock

Makes **about 6 cups**   Preparation time **10 minutes**   Cooking time **45 minutes**

2 onions, chopped

2 leeks, white part only, chopped

2 celery sticks, chopped

3 large carrots, chopped

1 small handful of parsley stems without leaves

2 bay leaves

2 thyme sprigs

12 black peppercorns

1   Put all of the ingredients and 6 cups water in a large saucepan. Bring almost to a boil, then turn the heat down to a low heat and simmer, covered, 40 minutes.

2   Let cool a little, then strain into a container and let cool completely. The stock will keep in the refrigerator up to 4 days or in the freezer up to 3 months.

basic recipes

Breakfasts

Breakfast in our home is either hectic and rushed or leisurely, depending on whether it's a weekday or the weekend. Whether you're running out the door or able to sit back and relax, here are recipes that will work brilliantly — and they're all delicious. Boost your energy levels for the day with Pineapple, Strawberry, and Passionfruit Smoothie, for example; or pack up some Brioche with Caramelized Peaches or Mango and Macadamia Muffins to take with you. Make pancake batter or bread the night before and tuck into Corn Pancakes or French Toast with Pears the next morning. Or cook up Spanish-Style Eggs and invite friends and family around to share them with you.

Apricot, Cranberry, and Goji Berry Granola, page 37 >

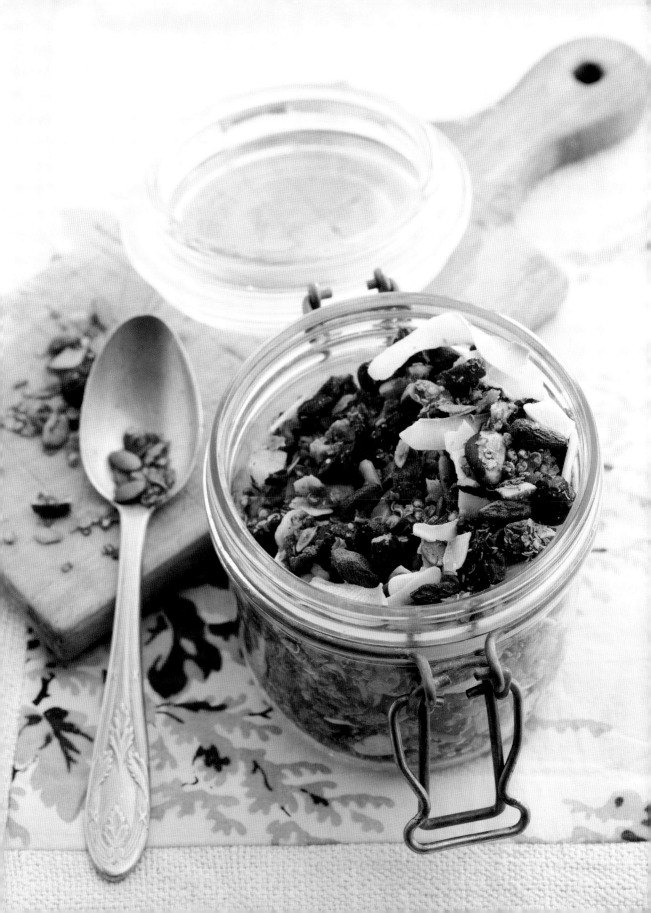

Smoothies make a wonderful start to the day. Full of vitamins, minerals, and protein, they give you energy and vitality.

Mango and Pomegranate Smoothie

Serves **4**   Preparation time **10 minutes**

2 large mangoes

1 cup pomegranate juice

1 cup unflavored soy yogurt

1 tablespoon flaxseeds

1   Using a sharp knife, carefully slice the mango down both sides, avoiding the seed. On the inside of each slice, cut the flesh into squares, cutting down to the peel but not piercing it, and scoop out with a spoon. Peel the remains of the mango and slice the flesh from the seed. Put all of the mango flesh in a blender or food processor.

2   Add all of the remaining ingredients and blend until smooth and creamy. Serve immediately.

Pineapple, Strawberry, and Passion Fruit Smoothie

Serves **4**   Preparation time **10 minutes**

1 pineapple

2⅔ cups strawberries, hulled

4 passion fruits, halved and seeds scooped out

1¾ cups coconut milk

2 tablespoons agave syrup

1   Trim the woody base and green top off the pineapple and, holding it upright, slice off and discard the skin, including the "eyes." Slice the flesh down the length of the fruit all around into long, thin slices, cutting around the core, then chop the flesh

2   Put the pineapple and all of the remaining ingredients in a blender or food processor and blend until smooth and creamy. Serve immediately.

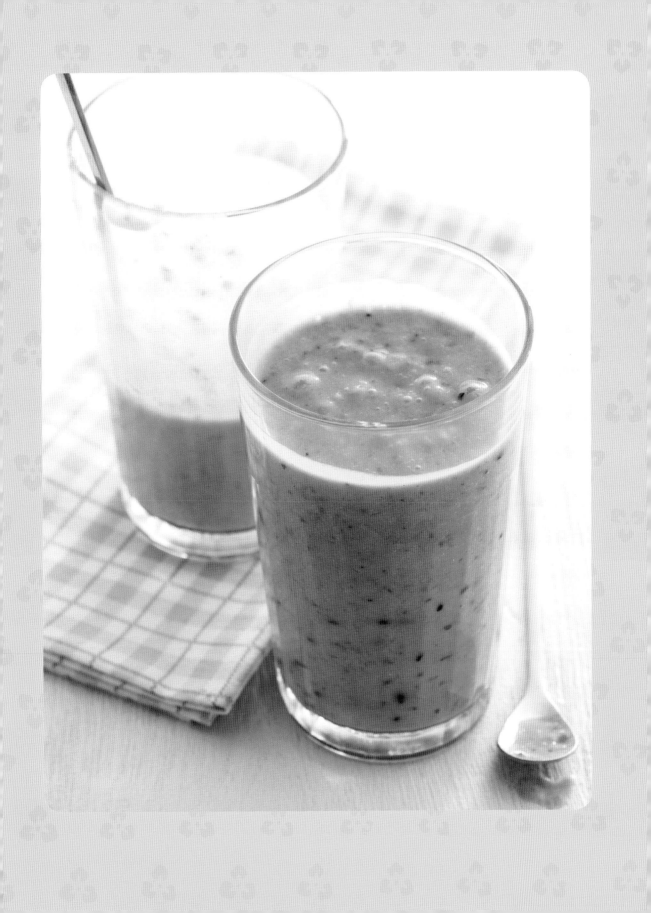

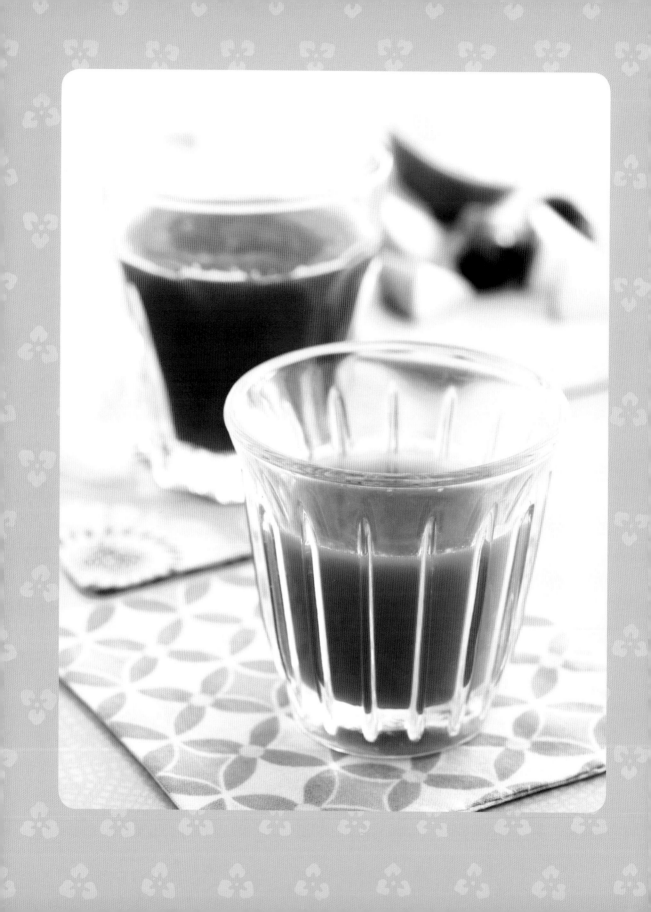

I adore juices! These recipes give you maximum nutrition along with either fruity, minty flavors or the taste of zingy ginger with sweet vegetables.

Apple, Blueberry, and Grape Juice

Serves **2**   Preparation time **5 minutes**

½ lime, halved

1 cup blueberries

2 large apples, quartered and stems removed

1 pound 2 ounces seedless grapes, stems removed

1 small handful of mint leaves

1   Scoop the flesh of the lime from the peel with a spoon and put it through an electric juicer. Juice all of the remaining ingredients and serve immediately.

Carrot, Pepper, Tomato, and Kiwi Juice

Serves **2**   Preparation time **5 minutes**

6 carrots, scrubbed and topped and tailed

1 red bell pepper, quartered

4 tomatoes, quartered

4 kiwi fruits, peeled and quartered

1-inch piece peeled ginger root

1   Put all of the ingredients through an electric juicer and serve immediately.

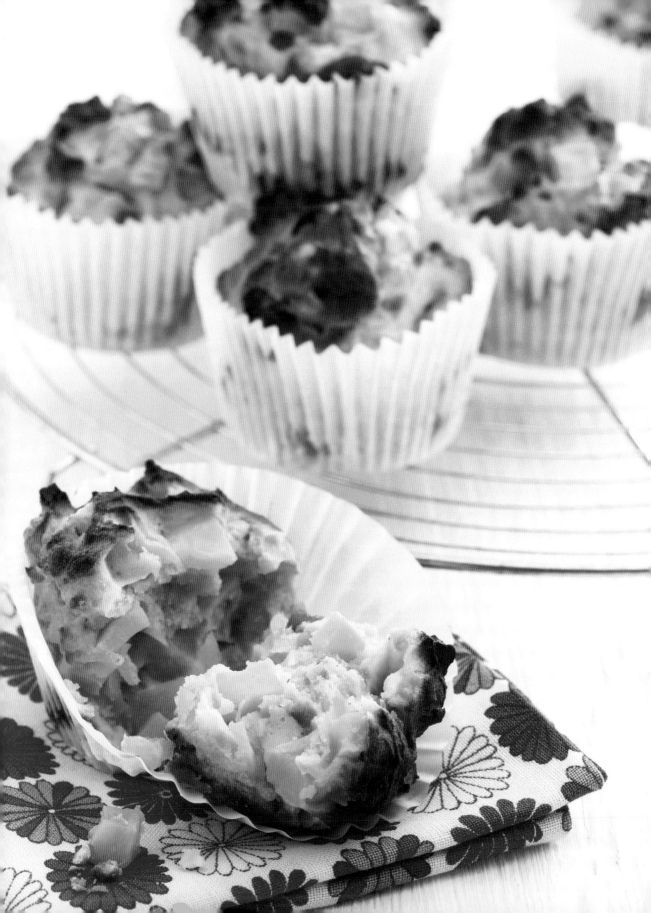

Here I'm using two of Australia's food heroes — macadamia nuts and mango. The first time I went to Sydney, some friends gave us boxes of gorgeously sweet mangoes and fresh macadamias. Great memories!

Mango and Macadamia Muffins

Makes **10**   Preparation time **15 minutes**   Cooking time **30 minutes**

1 large, very ripe mango

5 tablespoons dairy-free margarine, softened

½ cup less 2 tablespoons fruit sugar or granulated sugar

2 extra-large eggs

5 tablespoons plus 1 teaspoon unflavored soy yogurt

⅔ cup brown rice flour

heaped ½ cup chickpea flour

scant ½ cup corn flour

2 teaspoons gluten-free baking powder

½ teaspoon xanthan gum

3 tablespoons dried mango cut into small pieces

heaped ⅔ cup macadamia nuts, finely chopped

1   Preheat the oven to 350°F and put 10 paper muffin cases in a muffin pan. Using a sharp knife, carefully slice the mango down both sides, avoiding the seed. On the inside of each slice, cut the flesh into very small squares, cutting down to the peel but not piercing it, then scoop the flesh out with a spoon. Peel the remaining parts of the mangoes and cut the flesh off the seeds and cut into very small pieces. Set aside.

2   Put the dairy-free margarine and sugar in a large mixing bowl and, using an electric mixer, beat well until light and fluffy. Gradually beat in the eggs, one at a time, then beat in the soy yogurt.

3   Sift in the flours, gluten-free baking powder, and xanthan gum and stir quickly until mixed. Be careful not to overmix, and don't worry if there are some lumps in the batter. Stir in the fresh mango pieces, dried mango, and nuts, then spoon the batter into the muffin cases, filling each one about two-thirds full.

4   Bake 25 to 30 minutes until well risen, golden brown, and just firm to the touch, or until a skewer inserted into the middle comes out clean. Remove from the oven and eat the muffins warm or transfer them in their paper cases to a wire rack to cool.

breakfasts

My favorite combination of gluten-free flours is rice, chickpea, and corn because they balance each other in terms of taste and texture. In this recipe, I've used potato flour as well, to add moistness.

Brioche with Caramelized Peaches

Serves **4**   Preparation time **20 minutes, plus 4 hours rising**   Cooking time **30 minutes**

heaped ⅔ cup potato flour

heaped ½ cup chickpea flour

scant ½ cup corn flour

scant 1 cup brown rice flour

1 teaspoon fine sea salt

1 teaspoon xanthan gum

2 teaspoons active dry yeast

scant ¾ cup dairy-free margarine, chilled and cut into small pieces, plus extra for greasing

7 tablespoons soy milk

4 large eggs

6 tablespoons fruit sugar or granulated sugar

4 peaches, pitted and each sliced into 8 pieces

1 Sift the flours, salt, xanthan gum, and yeast into the bowl of a food processor with the dough blade attached and blend until mixed together. Add ⅔ cup of the dairy-free margarine and blend until the mixture resembles bread crumbs. Add the soy milk, 3 of the eggs, and 3 tablespoons of the sugar and process about 5 minutes to aerate the dough. Put the dough in a large bowl, cover with plastic wrap, and let rise 1 hour.

2 Grease a 12-hole muffin pan with dairy-free margarine. Stir the brioche dough thoroughly and pour evenly into the muffin pan. Cover loosely with plastic wrap and let rise 3 hours until light, puffy, and double in size.

3 Preheat the oven to 400°F. Beat the remaining egg and brush it over the brioches, using a pastry brush. Bake 20 minutes, or until golden brown. Let cool 2 to 3 minutes, then turn out of the pan and transfer to a wire rack before serving.

4 While the brioche are cooling, put the remaining margarine and sugar in a saucepan and heat over low heat until the dairy-free margarine melts and the sugar dissolves. Bring to a boil over high heat, then turn the heat down again to low and simmer 4 to 5 minutes until the mixture caramelizes slightly and becomes syrupy. Add the peaches to the saucepan and shake the pan to cover the peaches in the syrup. Cook 2 to 3 minutes until tender, continuing to shake the pan occasionally. Serve immediately with the brioche.

breakfasts

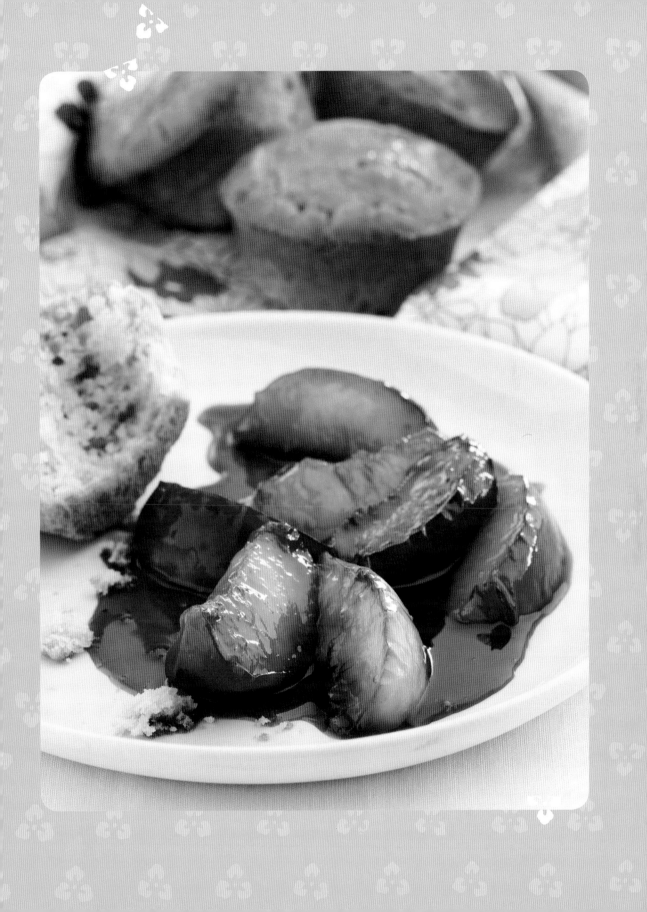

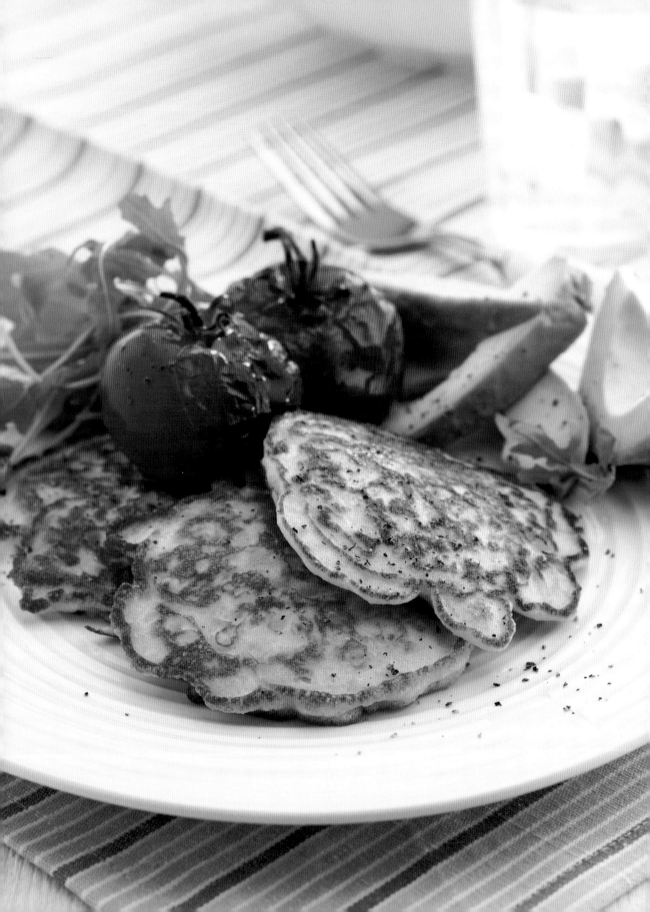

Frozen corn kernels are a wonderful staple ingredient. Sweet-flavored and filling, they work brilliantly in these pancakes.

Corn Pancakes

Makes **12 pancakes**   Preparation time **10 minutes**   Cooking time **30 minutes**

8 tomatoes

scant ½ cup corn kernels

scant ⅓ cup brown rice flour

scant ½ cup corn flour

a pinch of salt

1 teaspoon gluten-free baking powder

2 extra-large eggs

1 cup plus 2 tablespoons soy cream

1 tablespoon olive oil

freshly ground black pepper

2 avocados, peeled, pitted, and sliced, to serve

1 large handful of arugula leaves, to serve

1   Preheat the broiler to high. Broil the tomatoes 3 to 4 minutes until just starting to turn brown, then set aside.

2   Put the corn kernels in a steamer and steam over high heat 3 to 4 minutes until just tender.

3   Sift the flours, salt, and gluten-free baking powder into a large mixing bowl. Beat together the eggs and soy cream in another bowl. Make a well in the middle of the flour mixture and add the egg mixture. Beat slowly with a wooden spoon to draw in the flours to make a smooth batter. Stir in the corn kernels.

4   Heat the oil in a large, heavy-bottomed skillet over medium heat until hot. Pour 2 tablespoons of the batter into one half of the pan to make a pancake and then pour 2 more tablespoons into the other half. Cook 2 to 3 minutes on each side. or until golden.

5   Repeat with the remaining batter, adding more oil to the pan as needed. Stack the freshly cooked pancakes between sheets of nonstick baking parchment to prevent them from sticking together and to keep them warm. Note that the later pancakes will take less time on each side as the pan will have heated. Season with black pepper, then serve hot with the broiled tomatoes, avocados, and arugula leaves.

breakfasts

My daughter, Zoë, loves to be involved when I'm cooking. This is a great recipe to make with her because I can cook it with one hand while balancing her on my hip with the other.

French Toast with Pears

Serves **4**   Preparation time **5 minutes, plus making the bread**   Cooking time **30 minutes**

2 eggs

5 tablespoons plus 1 teaspoon soy milk

6 tablespoons fruit sugar or
   caster sugar

3 tablespoons dairy-free margarine

4 pears, peeled, cored and sliced lengthways

8 slices of White Bread (see page 14)

1   Put the eggs, soy milk, and scant 2 tablespoons of the sugar a large bowl. Beat well.

2   Put the remaining sugar and 2 tablespoons of the dairy-free margarine in a saucepan and heat over low heat until the margarine melts and the sugar dissolves. Bring to a boil over high heat, then turn the heat down again to low and simmer 4 to 5 minutes until the mixture caramelizes slightly and becomes syrupy.

3   Add the pears and shake the pan to cover them in the syrup. Cook 2 to 3 minutes until soft, continuing to shake the pan occasionally, then set aside.

4   Soak the bread in the egg mixture 2 minutes until completely soaked. Preheat the oven to 150°F. Put the remaining margarine in a skillet and heat over medium heat until it melts. Drain a couple of slices of the bread and fry 2 to 3 minutes on each side until golden brown. Remove from the pan and keep warm in the oven while you repeat with the remaining bread. Serve hot with the pears spooned over the French toast.

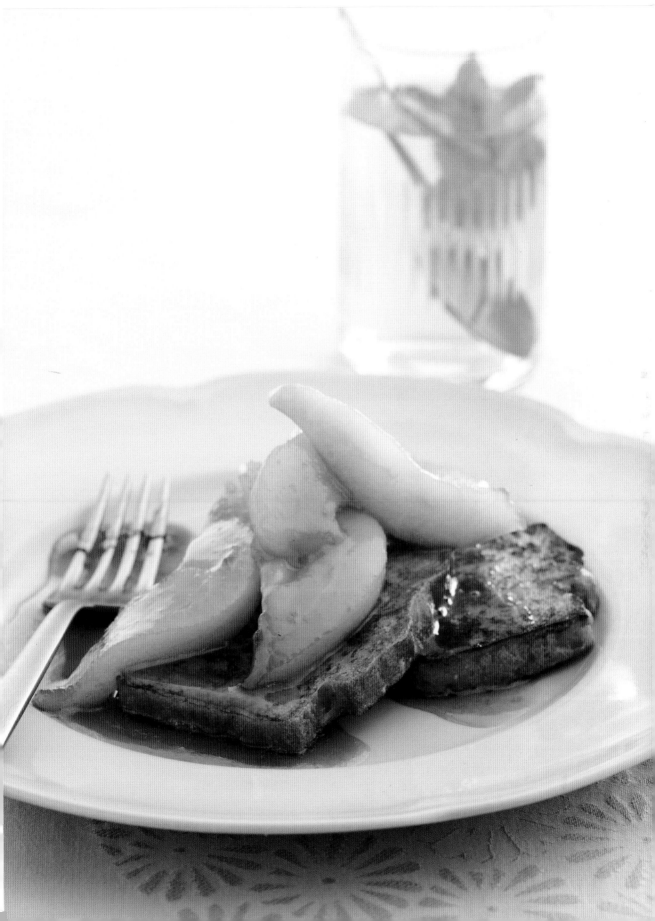

This muesli is a fantastic way to heap nutrients into your diet, including omega-3 fatty acids from the hemp and pumpkin seeds.

Muesli with Summer Fruit Compote

Makes **6 servings**   Preparation time **15 minutes**   Cooking time **35 minutes**

MUESLI:

¾ cup chopped hazelnuts

heaped 1 cup rice flakes

scant ½ cup buckwheat flakes

heaped ½ cup slivered almonds

1 cup toasted coconut flakes

2½ tablespoons pumpkin seeds

1 tablespoon hemp seeds

¾ cup unsulfured dried apricots, chopped

¼ cup pitted dates, chopped

2 tablespoons dried goji berries

soy yogurt, to serve

soy milk, to serve

SUMMER FRUIT COMPOTE:

8 apricots, pitted and quartered

8 plums, pitted and quartered

5 tablespoons fruit sugar or granulated sugar

1 cup blueberries

2⅔ cups strawberries, hulled

1   Preheat the oven to 350°F. To make the compote, put the apricots and plums in a medium-size baking dish, sprinkle the sugar over them, and bake 10 minutes. Gently stir in the blueberries and strawberries and bake 25 minutes longer, or until all the fruit is tender. Remove from the oven and let cool. Store in the refrigerator up to 3 days before serving.

2   To make the muesli, mix all of the ingredients together in a large mixing bowl.

3   Serve the muesli with the compote and with soy yogurt and soy milk, if desired. The muesli will keep in an airtight container up to 1 month.

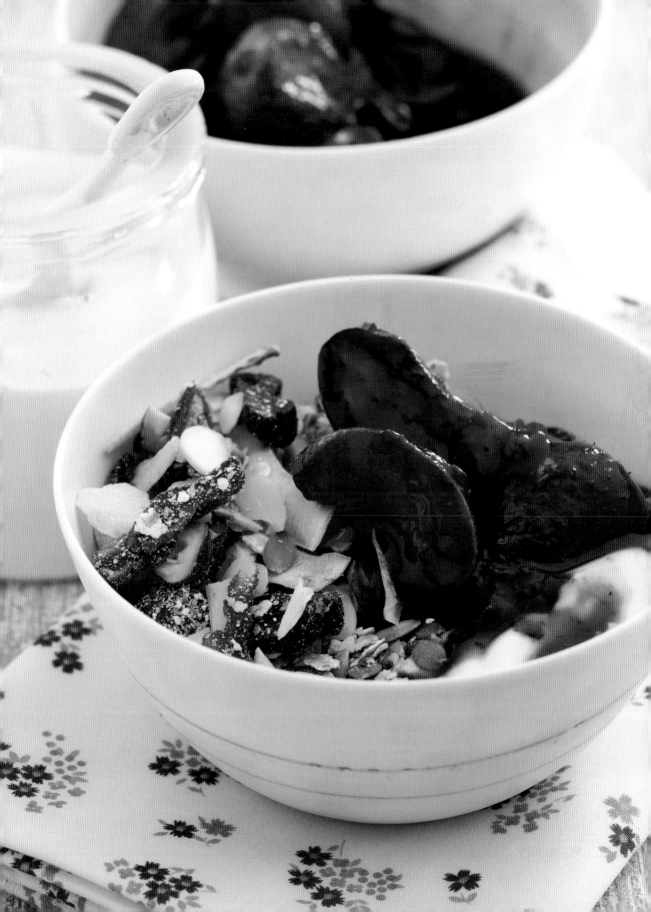

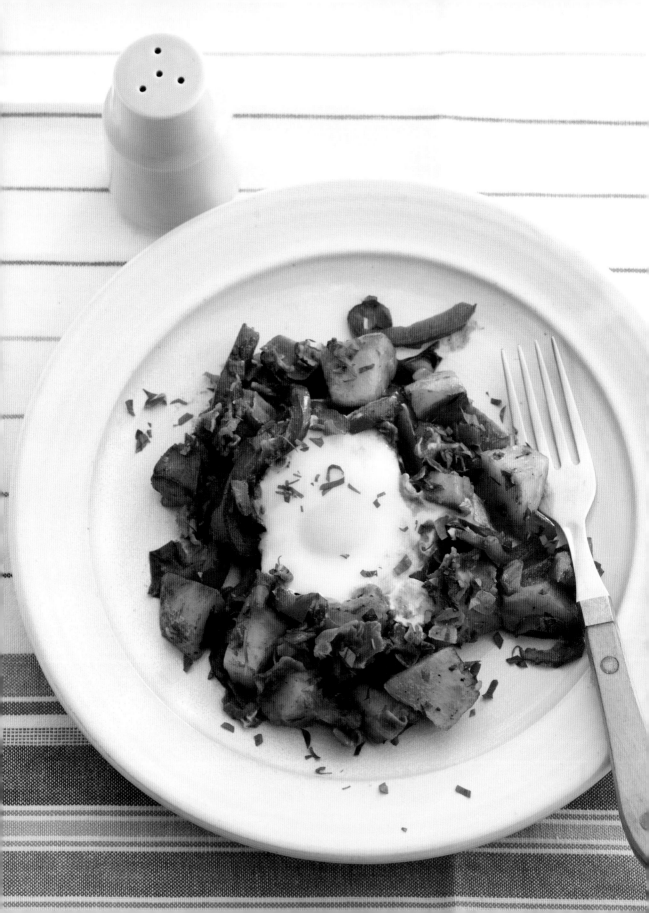

Classic ingredients combine here to make an extremely moreish dish that is perfect for a fill-you-up breakfast or brunch.

Spanish-Style Eggs

Serves 4   Preparation time **10 minutes**   Cooking time **35 minutes**

3 tablespoons olive oil

4 potatoes, cut into small chunks

1 large Spanish onion, chopped

2 red bell peppers, seeded and sliced

2 tablespoons tomato paste

8 tomatoes, chopped

scant ½ cup Vegetable Stock (see page 21) or vegetable stock made from gluten- and dairy-free bouillon powder

8 slices of Serrano ham or prosciutto, chopped

1 handful of chopped flat-leaf parsley leaves

4 eggs

sea salt and freshly ground black pepper

1   Heat the oil in a large, heavy-bottomed skillet and cook the potatoes over medium heat 8 to 10 minutes until starting to turn golden brown. Remove from the pan, using a slotted spoon, and transfer to a plate.

2   Add the onion to the pan and cook, stirring frequently, 2 to 3 minutes until just starting to turn golden. Add the peppers and cook, stirring frequently, 2 to 3 minutes longer, then stir in the tomato paste and season lightly with salt.

3   Add the tomatoes and stock and cook, covered, over low heat 10 minutes, or until the potatoes are tender. Stir occasionally and add a little more stock, if necessary. Gently stir in the ham and parsley.

4   With the back of a spoon, make 4 deep indentations in the mixture and crack an egg into each indentation. Cover again and cook 8 to 10 minutes until the egg whites are cooked through. Serve immediately.

breakfasts

Lunches

Trying to buy a gluten-and dairy-free lunch can often be a nightmare, and, even if you do find something, it's never as good as your own homemade food. Here you'll find nutritious meals you can eat at your desk, in the park, on the beach, or around your table at home. Take Tuna, Avocado, and Tomato Salsa Wraps to work, for example, or Shrimp, Fava Bean, and Avocado Bruschetta or Tomato Tart for a picnic in the sunshine. Put a smile on your kids' faces with Chicken and Sesame Nuggets or Chargrilled Pepper, Prosciutto, and Pine Nut Pizza; or make Spicy Pork Noodles or Crayfish and Asparagus Pasta for a delicious treat in the middle of the day.

Crayfish and Asparagus Pasta, page 65 >

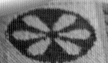

There's something very heartwarming about soup — and chicken soup in particular. This one is full of Asian flavors, with a kick from the chili.

Chicken and Coconut Soup

Serves **4**   Preparation time **15 minutes**   Cooking time **15 minutes**

2 lemongrass sticks, cut into thirds and bashed

1-inch piece of ginger root, peeled and coarsely chopped

1 red chili, seeded and coarsely chopped

2 shallots, coarsely chopped

2 kaffir lime leaves

4½ cups Chicken Stock (see page 20) or stock made from gluten- and dairy-free bouillon powder

1¾ cups coconut milk

2 boneless, skinless chicken breast halves, sliced into strips

2 cups chopped mushrooms

2 tablespoons Thai fish sauce

juice of ½ lime

1 large handful of cilantro leaves, chopped, to serve

1 Put the lemongrass, ginger, chili, and shallots in a mini food processor or spice mill. Pulse until finely chopped and the mixture forms a paste.

2 Put the paste in a large, heavy-bottomed saucepan and add the kaffir lime leaves, chicken stock, and coconut milk. Bring to a boil over high heat, then add the chicken, mushrooms, and fish sauce. Simmer over medium heat 10 minutes, or until the chicken is tender yet cooked through. To test that the chicken is cooked, remove a slice, prick with the tip of a sharp knife and check that the juice that runs out of it is clear, not pink.

3 Stir in the lime juice and serve immediately, sprinkled with the cilantro leaves.

lunches

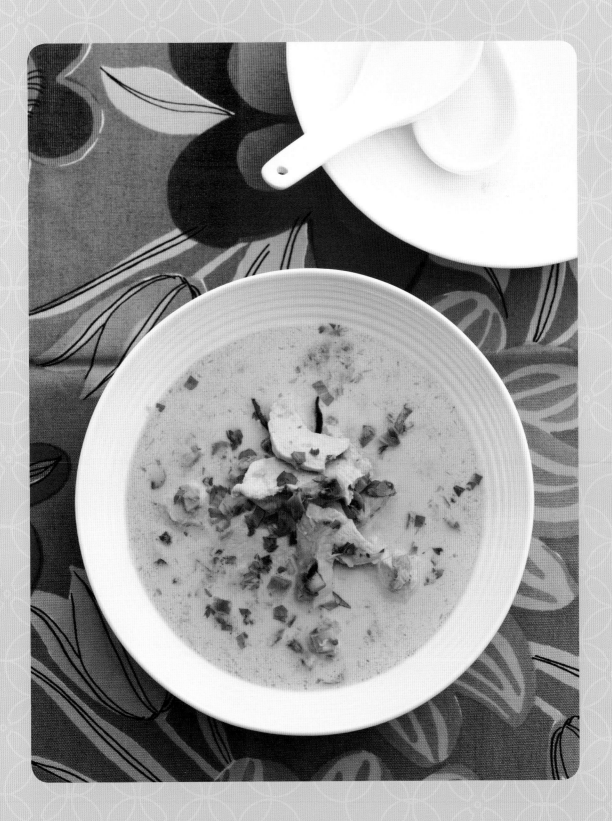

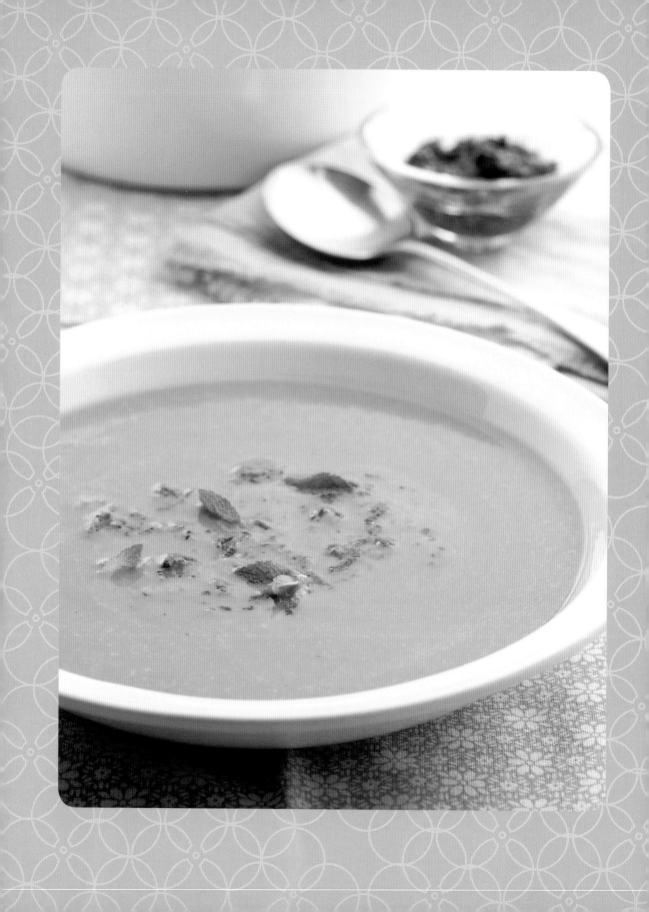

Mint and asparagus are a delicious combination — and the medicinal
qualities of mint can aid digestion and help digestive problems and IBS.

Asparagus Soup with Mint Pesto

Serves **4**   Preparation time **15 minutes**   Cooking time **30 minutes**

1 tablespoon olive oil

3 shallots, chopped

1 pound 2 ounces asparagus, woody ends
    removed and stalks roughly chopped

4½ cups Vegetable Stock (see page 21) or
    vegetable stock made from gluten- and
    dairy-free bouillon powder

6 large mint leaves, coarsely chopped

sea salt and freshly ground black pepper

MINT PESTO:

5 cups mint leaves, plus extra to decorate

⅓ cup pine nuts

2 garlic cloves

¼ cup olive oil

sea salt

1   Heat the oil in a large, heavy-bottomed saucepan over low heat. Add the shallots and cook,
    stirring occasionally, 2 to 3 minutes until golden. Stir in the asparagus and cook, stirring
    occasionally, 3 to 4 minutes until starting to soften.

2   Add the stock and chopped mint leaves and season lightly with salt and pepper. Bring to a
    boil over high heat, then turn the heat down to low and simmer, covered, 15 to 20 minutes.

3   Meanwhile, make the pesto. Rinse and carefully pat the mint dry in a clean dish towel.
    Heat a dry, heavy-bottomed skillet over medium heat. Add the pine nuts and toast,
    stirring frequently, until just starting to turn golden. Remove from the heat and transfer
    to a food processor.

4   Add the mint leaves and garlic and start to blend. With the motor running, add the oil
    and blend until the mixture forms a thick, dense sauce. Transfer to a bowl and season with
    salt to taste.

5   Blend the soup until smooth. Stir in a large spoonful of the pesto, sprinkle with mint leaves,
    and serve. The remaining pesto will keep in the refrigerator 1 to 2 days, or in the freezer
    up to 3 months.

Mushrooms always conjure up lovely memories of picking them with my father when I was young. Here I've used both fresh and dried ones for a richer flavor, as well as hazelnuts to add creamy thickness to the soup.

Wild Mushroom and Hazelnut Cream Soup

Serves **4**   Preparation time **35 minutes, plus at least 12 hours soaking**   Cooking time **30 minutes**

heaped ⅓ cup blanched hazelnuts

¾ ounce dried porcini mushrooms

2 tablespoons olive oil

1 onion, chopped

2 garlic cloves, crushed

1 pound mixed wild mushrooms, such
   as chanterelle, porcini, and oyster, washed
   and sliced

1 cup plus 2 tablespoons Vegetable Stock
   (see page 21) or vegetable stock made from
   gluten- and dairy-free bouillon powder

1 handful of parsley leaves, chopped

sea salt and freshly ground black pepper

1 Put the hazelnuts in a bowl, cover with cold water, and let soak overnight, or at least 12 hours, then drain and rinse well.

2 Put the dried mushrooms in a bowl and cover with 2 cups boiling water. Let soak 20 minutes, then remove with a slotted spoon and set aside. Strain the liquid into a clean bowl and set aside.

3 Heat the oil in a large, heavy-bottomed saucepan over low heat. Add the onion and cook, stirring occasionally, 2 to 3 minutes until golden, then add the garlic and cook, stirring, 30 seconds longer. Gently stir in the mushrooms and cook 3 to 4 minutes, continuing to stir occasionally. Add the stock and reserved mushroom liquid and season lightly with salt and pepper. Bring to a boil over high heat, then turn down the heat to low and simmer, covered, 15 to 20 minutes. Stir in the parsley and simmer 2 minutes longer.

4 Meanwhile, put the hazelnuts in a food processor or blender and add ⅓ cup water. Blend 10 minutes, or until very smooth. Transfer to a small bowl.

5 Blend the soup until smooth. Serve with a spoonful of the hazelnut cream stirred in each bowl. The remaining hazelnut cream will keep in the refrigerator up to 3 days, or in the freezer up to 3 months.

Sesame seeds are a great alternative to bread crumbs. They are exceptionally high in calcium, making these nuggets a super-healthy option for kids.

Chicken Sesame Nuggets

Serves **4** Preparation time **15 minutes, plus at least 2 hours marinating** Cooking time **20 minutes**

4 skinless, boneless chicken breast halves, sliced
  into short strips
1 cup sesame seeds

MARINADE:
½ cup honey
2 tablespoons tamari soy sauce
16 scallions, finely sliced
2-inch piece of ginger root, peeled and finely
  chopped

1   Put the chicken in a nonreactive baking dish. Mix together all of the ingredients for the marinade in a bowl and pour the mixture over the chicken. Cover and let marinate in the refrigerator at least 2 to 3 hours, or overnight.

2   Preheat the oven to 350°F and line two baking trays with baking parchment. Put the sesame seeds in a sandwich bag, remove the chicken pieces from the marinade and put them in the bag. Gently shake until all of the pieces are covered in seeds. Put the chicken on the baking trays and discard any remaining seeds.

3   Put the dish with the marinade in the oven, uncovered, along with the chicken. Bake 15 to 20 minutes until the chicken is cooked through. Serve with a little of the marinade sauce poured over the nuggets.

lunches

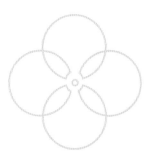

Lentils are a pantry essential that provides a great source of sustained energy. Combined with the delicious aromas and flavors from the rosemary, garlic, pancetta, and chicken here, they make a gorgeous meal.

Rosemary Chicken Skewers with Puy Lentils

Serves **4**   Preparation time **30 minutes, plus at least 12 hours soaking and 1 hour marinating**
Cooking time **55 minutes**

1 cup Puy lentils

2 garlic cloves, peeled but left whole, plus
    1 crushed

¼ cup olive oil

2 large skinless, boneless chicken breast halves,
    cut into bite-size pieces

4 ounces pancetta

3 shallots, finely chopped

2½ cups Chicken Stock (see page 20)
    or stock made from gluten- and dairy-free
    bouillon powder

4 long rosemary sprigs, lower leaves removed

sea salt and freshly ground black pepper

1 Rinse the lentils thoroughly and put them in a large bowl. Cover with water and let soak overnight, or at least 12 hours, then drain, rinse well, and drain again.

2 Put the whole garlic and 3 tablespoons of the oil in a mini food processor or spice mill and blend 2 to 3 minutes until smooth and thick. Put the chicken in a shallow dish, pour the garlic mixture over the top, and stir well to coat the chicken pieces. Cover and let marinate in the refrigerator 1 hour, or until needed.

3 Heat the remaining oil in a skillet over medium heat. Add the pancetta and fry 5 to 6 minutes until crisp. Using a slotted spoon, transfer the pancetta to a heavy-bottomed saucepan and set aside. Add the shallots to the skillet and fry, stirring occasionally, 2 minutes, or until starting to turn golden, then add the crushed garlic and fry 30 seconds longer. Add the mixture to the saucepan, along with all the fat from the skillet, then add the lentils and stock. Bring to a boil over high heat, then the heat down to low and simmer, covered, 45 minutes, or until soft. When cooked, drain off any excess liquid and season with salt and pepper.

4 Meanwhile, soak the rosemary sprigs in cold water 20 minutes and preheat the broiler to high. Thread the chicken pieces onto the rosemary sprigs and put on the broiler pan. When the lentils have been cooking for about 25 minutes, broil the skewers 20 minutes, turning every 5 minutes, until cooked through and light brown. Serve with the lentils.

lunches

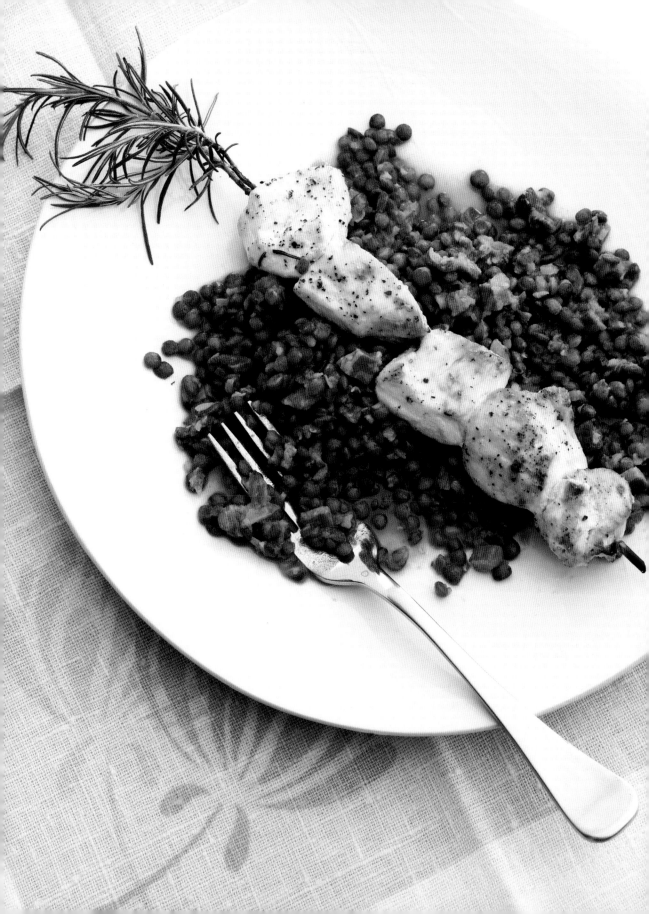

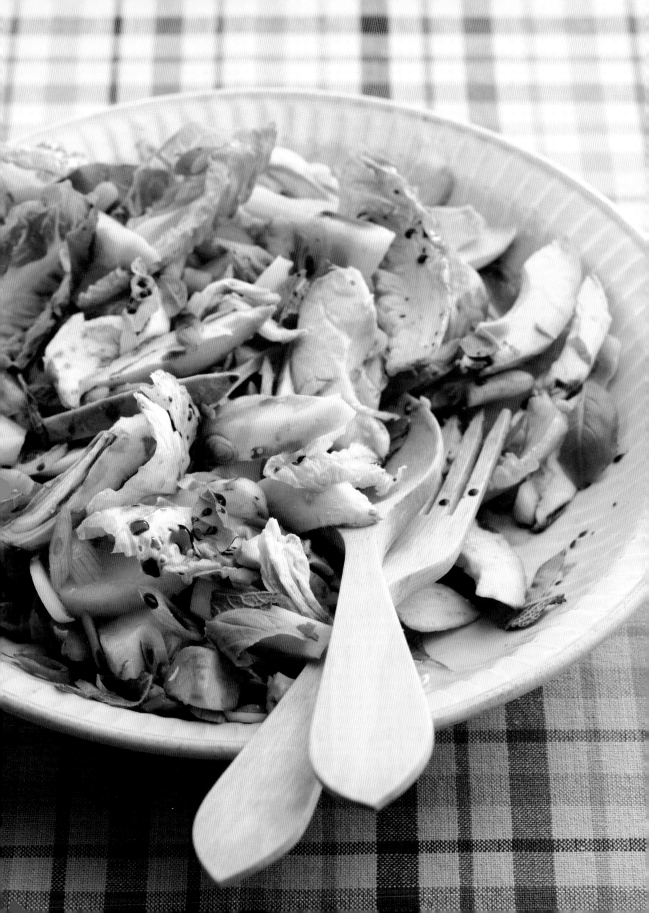

A very simple summer salad—but full of freshness from the herbs, sweetness from the mango, and deep rich flavor from the balsamic vinegar.

Chicken and Mango Salad

Serves **4**   Preparation time **15 minutes**   Cooking time **25 minutes**

4 skinless, boneless chicken breast halves

5 tablespoons olive oil

2 mangoes

4 avocados, peeled, seeded, and sliced

12 scallions, finely sliced

4 hearts of lettuces, leaves separated

1 handful of basil leaves, chopped

1 handful of mint leaves, chopped

¼ cup balsamic vinegar

1   Preheat the oven to 350°F. Put the chicken breasts in a baking dish, drizzle with 1 tablespoon of the oil, and cover. Bake 20 to 25 minutes until cooked through. To test that the chicken is cooked, prick with the tip of a sharp knife and check that the juice that runs out of it is clear, not pink. Remove from the oven and let cool completely.

2   With a sharp knife, carefully slice the mangoes down both sides, avoiding the seed. On the inside of each slice, cut the flesh into slices, cutting down to the peel but not piercing it, then carefully scoop out with a spoon. Peel the remaining parts of the mangoes and cut the flesh off the seeds in slices. Put the mango in a large salad bowl and add the avocados, scallions, lettuces, and herbs.

3   Either chop or tear the cooled chicken into bite-size pieces and add it to the bowl. Drizzle with the vinegar and remaining oil and toss gently but thoroughly. Serve immediately.

A nutrient-dense dish that's bursting with antioxidants, beta-carotene, vitamins, and minerals, as well as full-on flavors. Here I've used rice noodles, but you can use glass noodles instead.

Spicy Pork Noodles

Serves **4**   Preparation time **20 minutes, plus 30 minutes marinating**   Cooking time **15 minutes**

1 pound 4 ounces pork tenderloin, cut into strips

9 ounces rice noodles

6 scallions, white part only, finely sliced

2 cups sugar-snap peas

4 cups bean sprouts

1 red bell pepper, seeded and sliced

1 yellow bell pepper, seeded and sliced

1 bok choy, cut into thirds, stems and leaves
    separated

⅓ cup sesame seeds, to serve

1 handful of cilantro leaves, chopped, to serve

MARINADE:

2 garlic cloves

1 red chili, seeded and cut into large pieces

2 lemongrass stalks, cut into large pieces

2 tablespoons tamari soy sauce

1 tablespoon toasted sesame oil

1 tablespoon olive oil

1 tablespoon Thai fish sauce

1 tablespoon rice wine vinegar

1 tablespoon agave syrup

1 tablespoon Chinese five-spice powder

1   To make the marinade, put the garlic, chili, and lemongrass in a mini food processor or spice mill and blend until finely chopped. Put the mixture and the remaining ingredients for the marinade in a shallow, nonreactive bowl and mix well. Add the pork to the marinade and stir well, making sure the pork is covered in the marinade. Cover and chill in the refrigerator at least 30 minutes, or overnight.

2   Put the noodles in a large heatproof bowl, cover with boiling water, and let stand 5 minutes, or until soft. Drain well.

3   Heat a wok or large skillet over high heat. Add the pork, marinade, and scallions and stir-fry 5 minutes, then add the sugar-snap peas, bean sprouts, peppers, and bok choy stems. Stir-fry 5 minutes longer, then add the bok choy leaves. Stir-fry 2 to 3 minutes longer until the pork is cooked through and the vegetables are cooked but still slightly crunchy. Stir in the noodles and serve sprinkled with the sesame seeds and cilantro leaves.

lunches

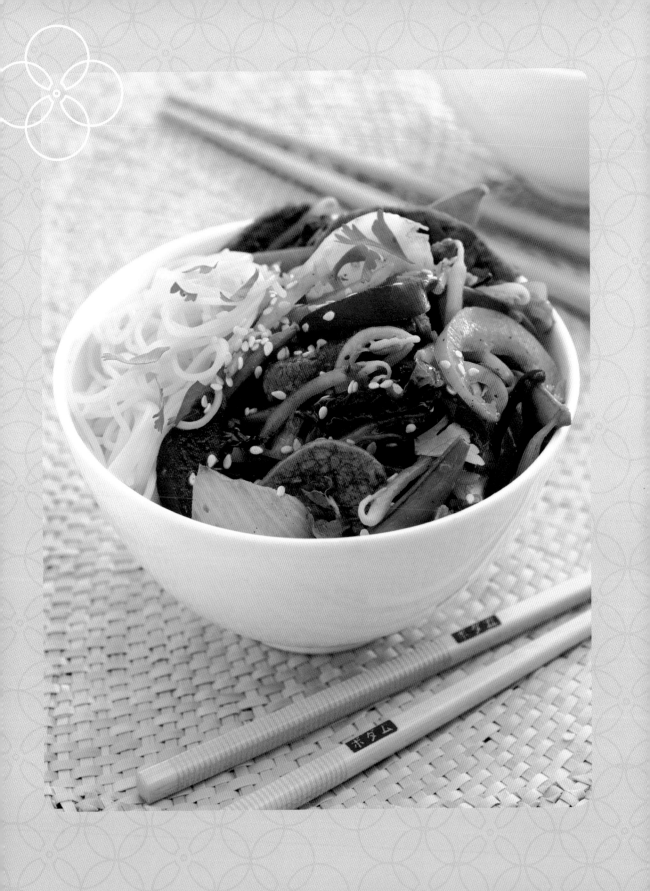

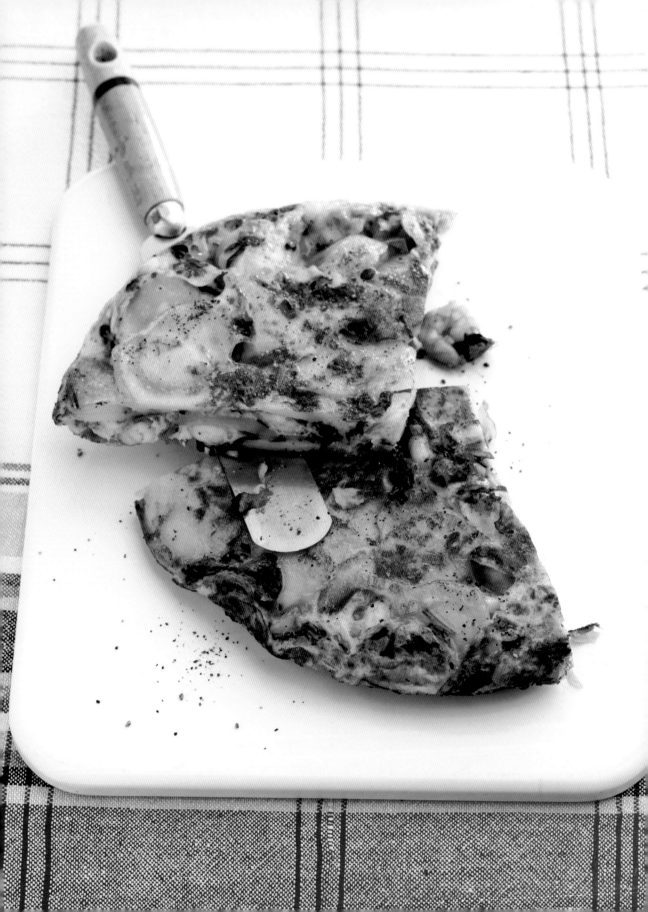

This is a fantastically versatile dish. You can eat it hot at home or pack it up into a chilled lunchbox for work or a picnic.

Spinach and Prosciutto Tortilla

Serves **4**   Preparation time **15 minutes**   Cooking time **30 minutes**

1 cup plus 2 tablespoons olive oil

2 large potatoes, thinly sliced

1 large Spanish onion, finely chopped

2 garlic cloves, crushed

8 slices of prosciutto, chopped

8 ounces spinach leaves, chopped

6 extra-large eggs

8 ounces raw shrimp

sea salt and freshly ground black pepper

1 Heat the oil in a large, nonstick skillet over medium heat. Add half of the potato slices and cook, stirring occasionally, 5 to 6 minutes until soft and starting to turn golden brown. Remove from the pan with a slotted spoon, set aside, and repeat with the remaining potato slices.

2 Add the onion to the oil and cook, stirring occasionally, 2 to 3 minutes until starting to turn golden. Add the garlic and fry 30 seconds, then remove the mixture from the pan with a slotted spoon and discard the oil. Return the onion and garlic mixture to the pan and add the prosciutto and spinach. Cook, stirring frequently, 2 minutes, or until the spinach starts to wilt.

3 Beat the eggs together in a bowl and season lightly with salt and pepper. Add the shrimp and the potatoes to the skillet and pour in the egg mixture. Stir gently to mix well, then cook about 10 minutes, or until the tortilla turns golden on the bottom. Remove the pan from the heat, hold a large plate upside-down over the pan and turn the pan over so the tortilla falls out onto the plate. Slide the inverted tortilla back into the skillet and cook the other side 5 minutes, or until golden brown on the bottom. Serve warm.

Thought you couldn't eat pizza? Think again! This gluten-free and dairy-free pizza has a thick crust that is deliciously crunchy and crispy on the edges.

Chargrilled Pepper, Prosciutto, and Pine Nut Pizza

Serves **2**   Preparation time **25 minutes, plus 30 minutes rising**   Cooking time **15 minutes**

3 tablespoons pine nuts

generous ⅓ cup tomato puree

2 tablespoons tomato paste

1 cup drained jarred or canned peppers in oil,
    cut into strips

2 ounces prosciutto, thinly sliced

10 cherry tomatoes, halved

10 large basil leaves, torn into small pieces

⅓ to ⅔ cup soy cheese, shaved

PIZZA DOUGH:

½ cup brown rice flour, plus extra for dusting

scant 1 cup chickpea flour

¼ cup corn flour

scant ½ teaspoon xanthan gum

½ teaspoon salt

1 teaspoon active dry yeast

2 tablespoons olive oil

1   To make the pizza dough, sift the flours, xanthan gum, salt, and yeast into a large mixing bowl and whisk to mix together. Add the olive oil and mix again, then add scant ½ cup warm water and, using either a wooden spoon or your hands, mix well to form a soft dough. Cover the bowl with plastic wrap and let stand at room temperature 30 minutes.

2   Preheat the oven to 425°F and line a baking sheet with parchment paper. Lightly toast the pine nuts in a dry frying pan over medium heat for 1 minute, stirring.

3   Turn the dough out again onto a lightly floured surface and knead a little, then shape it into a ball. Flatten the dough slightly, roll it out into a large circle about ¼ inch thick and neaten the edge, using a sharp knife. Transfer the dough to the baking sheet.

4   Put the tomato puree and tomato paste in a bowl and mix well, then spread it over the pizza base and scatter the peppers, prosciutto, cherry tomatoes and basil over the top. Bake 12 minutes until the crust is starting to turn brown and the tomato sauce is bubbling. Remove the pizza from the oven and sprinkle the cheese and pine nuts over the top, then return to the oven 3 to 4 minutes longer until the cheese starts to melt. Serve immediately.

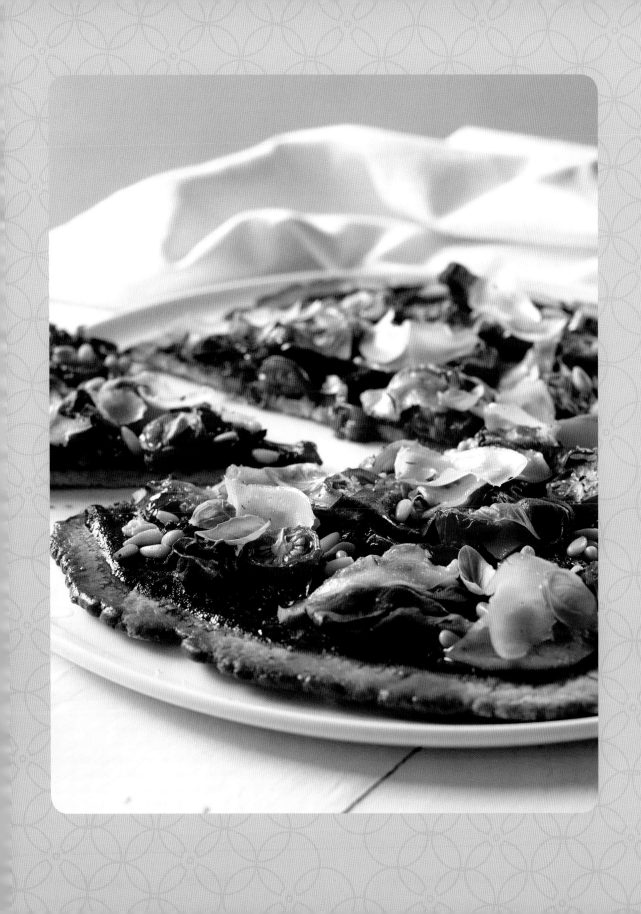

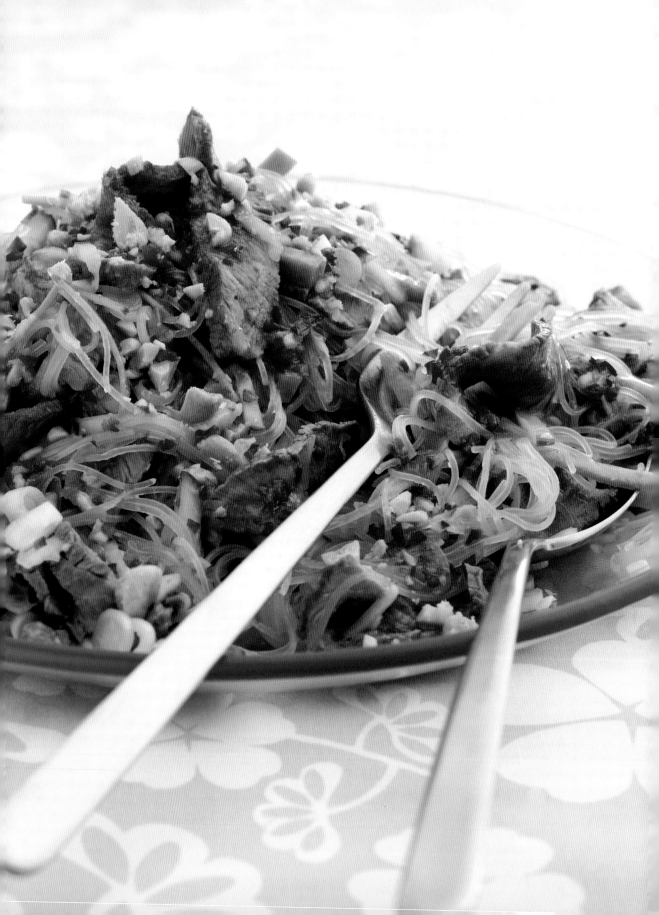

Ume plum vinegar, made from umeboshi plums, has a zesty flavor that's a wonderful alternative to citrus or other vinegars. Here it gives a sharp, tangy flavor to the noodles and beef salad.

Asian Beef Salad with Glass Noodles

Serves **4**   Preparation time **25 minutes**   Cooking time **5 minutes**

8 ounces dried glass noodles (mung bean
    vermicelli)

1 tablespoon olive oil

2 large sirloin steaks

1 large handful of cilantro leaves, chopped

1 handful of mint leaves, chopped

1 cucumber, cut into matchsticks

3 carrots, cut into matchsticks

12 scallions, white part only, finely sliced

2 Little Gem lettuces, torn into bite-size pieces

sea salt

⅔ cup peanuts, chopped, to serve

UME PLUM DRESSING:

2 chilies, seeded and chopped into large chunks

2 garlic cloves, crushed

juice of 1 lime

2 tablespoons agave syrup

2 tablespoons ume plum vinegar

2 tablespoons Thai fish sauce

3 tablespoons olive oil

1   To make the dressing, put the chilies in a mini food processor or spice mill and blend until finely chopped. Transfer to a pitcher and add all of the remaining ingredients for the dressing. Whisk together and set aside.

2   Put the glass noodles in a large heatproof bowl, cover with boiling water, and let stand 5 minutes, or until translucent. Drain well.

3   Heat the oil in a skillet or griddle pan over medium heat. Season the steaks lightly with salt and fry 2 minutes on each side, or until brown on the outside but still pink in the middle. Slice each steak into thin strips and put them in a large salad bowl. Add the noodles and all of the remaining ingredients, except the peanuts. Pour the dressing over the salad and toss well. Sprinkle with the peanuts and serve.

Tuna is a brilliant source of omega-3 fats. Here it's served with an avocado and tomato salsa and wrapped in warm tortillas. You'll never want to go back to dull, dry sandwiches again!

Tuna, Avocado, and Tomato Salsa Wraps

Serves **4**   Preparation time **15 minutes, plus making the tortillas**   Cooking time **5 minutes**

4 tomatoes, diced

6 scallions, finely sliced

1 large red chili, seeded and finely chopped

1 large handful of cilantro leaves, chopped

juice of 1 lime

3 avocados, peeled, pitted, and roughly mashed

4 tuna steaks

1 tablespoon olive oil

1 recipe quantity warm Corn Tortillas
  (see page 17)

8 large spinach leaves

sea salt

1   To make the salsa, mix the tomatoes, scallions, chili, cilantro leaves, and lime juice together in a large bowl and set aside. Season the avocado lightly with salt.

2   Heat a skillet or griddle pan over high heat. Brush the tuna lightly on each side with the oil, season lightly with salt, and cook 2 to 3 minutes on each side until brown on the outside but slightly pink in the middle. Remove from the pan and let rest 2 to 3 minutes, then slice into thin strips.

3   Spread a couple spoonfuls of avocado down the middle of each tortilla. Cover with 1 spinach leaf, a few tuna strips, and a couple spoonfuls of the salsa mixture. Roll up the tortillas, using baking parchment to hold the tortilla firm, and cut each one in half diagonally. Use toothpicks to secure the tortillas, if necessary, and serve.

lunches

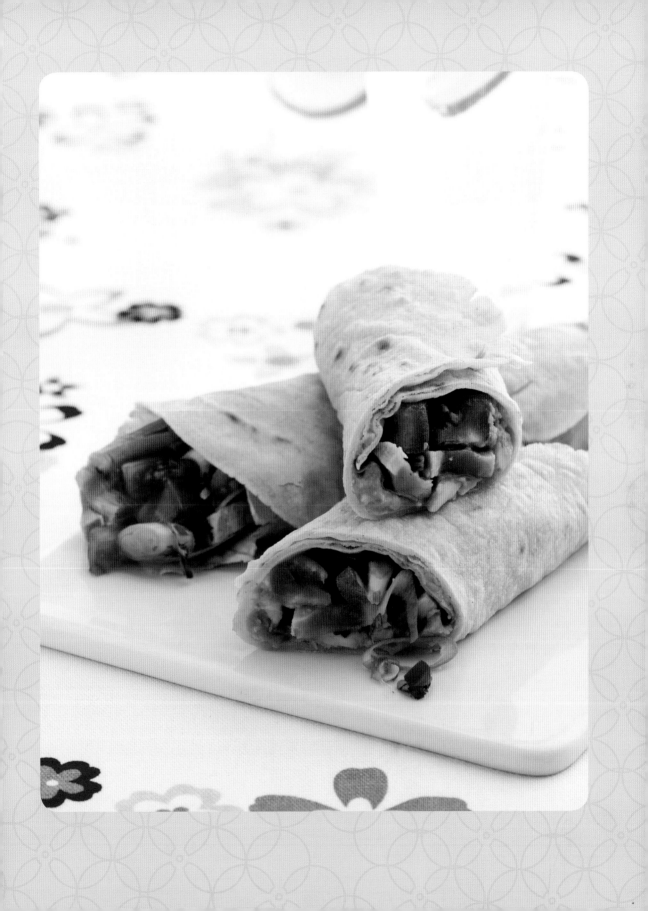

Cornstarch is a gem of an ingredient. You can use it to thicken sauces and desserts and combine it with spices to make a delicious coating for fish and seafood, especially the squid in this recipe.

Salt and Pepper Squid

Serves **4**   Preparation time **15 minutes**   Cooking time **15 minutes**

14 ounces dressed baby squid

1 teaspoon Sichuan peppercorns

1 teaspoon sea salt

¼ teaspoon Chinese five-spice powder

¼ cup cornstarch

2 cups canola oil

lime wedges, to serve

DIPPING SAUCE:

½-inch piece of ginger root, peeled and coarsely chopped

1 red chili, deseeded and coarsely chopped

1 tablespoon Thai fish sauce

1 tablespoon tamari soy sauce

2 tablespoons honey

juice of 1 lime

1 small handful of cilantro leaves

1 Put all of the ingredients for the dipping sauce in a mini food processor or spice mill and blend until smooth.

2 Cut the tentacles off the squid and set aside. Using a sharp knife, cut down one side of the squid tubes and open out flat. Score on the inside with a diamond pattern and pat the tubes and tentacles dry with paper towels.

3 Heat a dry, heavy-bottomed skillet over low heat. Add the Sichuan peppercorns and cook 2 to 3 minutes until slightly brown, stirring continuously so they do not burn. Remove from the heat and transfer to a mini food processor or spice mill. Add the salt and grind to a fine powder, then transfer to a small bowl and stir in the five-spice powder and cornstarch.

4 Dip the squid tubes and tentacles in the flour mixture, coating them well, then put them on a plate.

5 Heat the oil in a deep skillet or wok over high heat until very hot. Working in batches to avoid overcrowding the pan, deep-fry the squid 3 minutes, or until light golden. Remove from the oil with a slotted spoon and drain on paper towels. Serve immediately with the dipping sauce.

lunches

My husband loves this! The clean sharp tastes of the chili and lemon combine with the herbs and seafood to make a seriously good dish.

Crayfish and Asparagus Pasta

Serves **4**   Preparation time **15 minutes**   Cooking time **15 minutes**

2 shallots, halved

1 red chili, halved and seeded

2 garlic cloves

3 strips of lemon zest

7 tablespoons olive oil

12 ounces gluten-free pasta

12 ounces asparagus, woody ends removed and
   stalks cut into thirds

½ cup Fish Stock (see page 20) or stock made
   from gluten- and dairy-free bouillon powder

12 ounces crayfish tails

1 large handful of flat-leaf parsley leaves,
   chopped

juice of ½ lemon, plus lemon quarters, to serve

sea salt and freshly ground black pepper

1   Put the shallots, chili, garlic, and lemon zest in a mini food processor or spice mill and
    blend until finely chopped, making sure the zest is coarsely chopped.

2   Bring a large saucepan of water to a boil and stir in 1 tablespoon of the oil. Add the pasta
    and cook over medium heat 8 to 10 minutes, or according to the directions on the package,
    until soft. Make sure you stir occasionally so the pasta doesn't stick. Drain and rinse well
    with freshly boiled water, then drain again.

3   Meanwhile, in a large, heavy-bottomed saucepan, heat 4 tablespoons of the remaining oil
    over medium heat. Add the shallot mixture and fry, stirring, about 1 minute until starting
    to turn golden. Add the asparagus and stir well. Fry for another minute, then add the fish
    stock. Cook, covered, 4 minutes, then add the crayfish. Cook 2 minutes longer until the
    asparagus is tender but still slightly crunchy.

4   Add the cooked pasta to the saucepan and mix well. Add the parsley, lemon juice, and the
    remaining 2 tablespoons of olive oil. Season with salt and pepper and serve immediately
    with lemon quarters for squeezing over.

Make the most of delicious, fresh fava beans when you can. If they're not available, though, you can either use frozen fava beans or edamame beans.

Shrimp, Fava Bean, and Avocado Bruschetta

Serves **4**   Preparation time **15 minutes, plus making the bread**   Cooking time **5 minutes**

2 pounds 4 ounces fresh fava beans, podded
   (or about 1½ cups frozen)

1 avocado

12 ounces cooked, shelled shrimp, chopped

1 tablespoon finely chopped mint leaves, plus
   a few mint sprigs for cooking

1 tablespoon finely chopped basil leaves

1 small handful of cilantro leaves,
   finely chopped

1 tablespoon lime juice

2 tablespoons olive oil

scant ½ teaspoon crushed chili flakes

2 or 3 garlic cloves, peeled

12 to 16 slices of White Bread (see page 14),
   toasted

sea salt

1   Put the beans and mint sprigs in a steamer and steam, covered, over high heat 4 to 5 minutes until tender. Remove and discard the mint.

2   Rinse the beans under cold running water, then drain well and transfer to a bowl. Remove and discard the skins from the beans by squeezing the skins until the beans pop out. Mash the beans coarsely. Peel the avocado, remove and discard the pit, then mash the flesh coarsely and stir it into the beans. Add the shrimp, chopped herbs, lime juice, olive oil, and chili flakes and mix well. Season to taste with salt.

3   Rub the garlic onto the toasted bread slices and top with a spoonful of the shrimp mixture. Serve immediately.

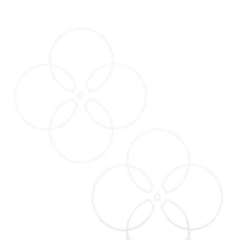

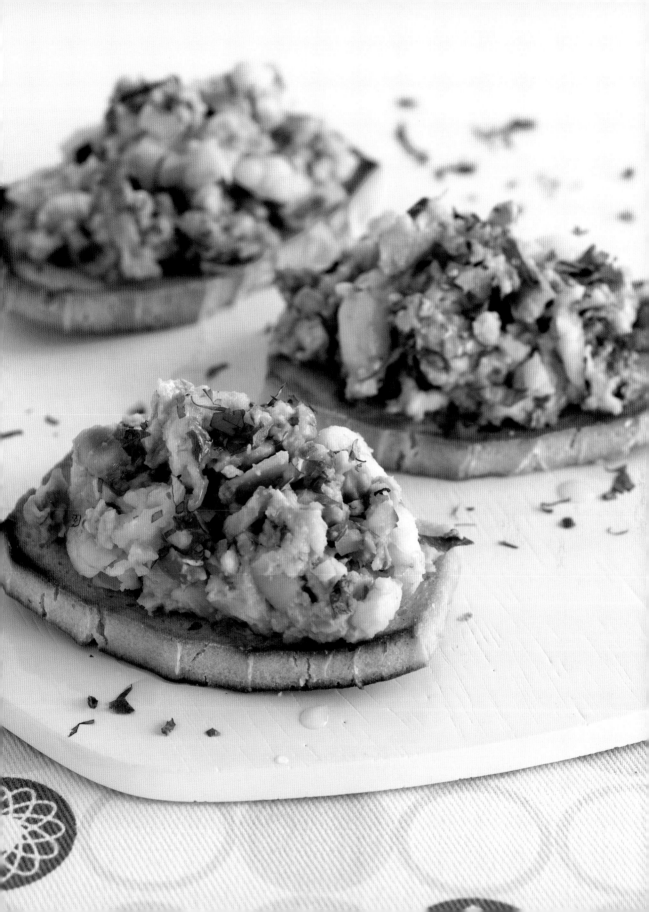

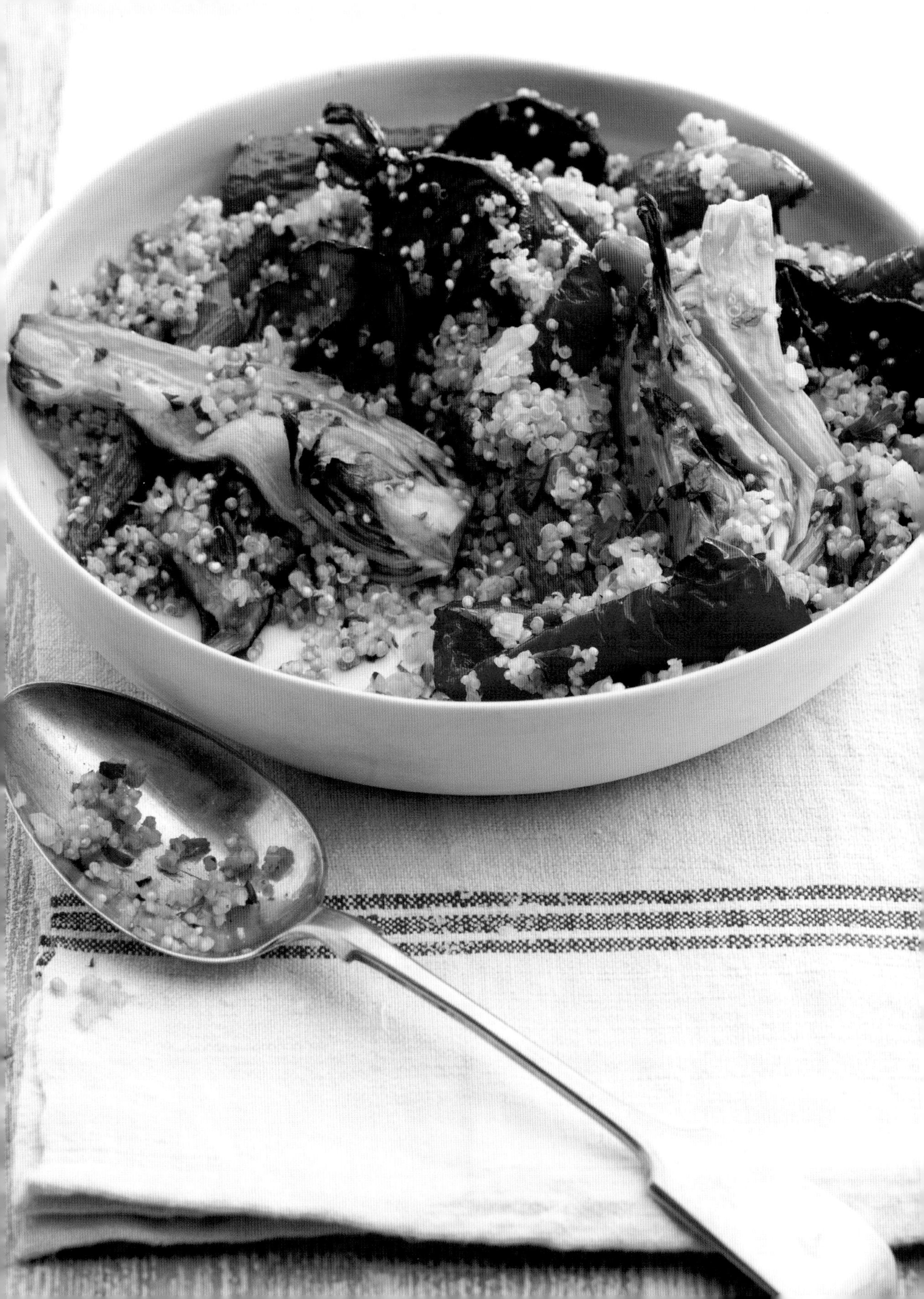

Quinoa contains all eight essential amino acids, as well as high quantities of calcium and magnesium, so it's wonderful to include in your repertoire. Frying the quinoa before adding the water enhances the taste and texture.

Roasted Vegetables and Quinoa

Serves **4**   Preparation time **15 minutes**   Cooking time **45 minutes**

20 small carrots

10 small beets, halved

3 fennel bulbs, fronds removed, and quartered

2 eggplants, quartered

2 red bell peppers, seeded and quartered

½ cup olive oil

1 large onion, chopped

1½ cups quinoa

2 teaspoons ground cumin

2 teaspoons ground coriander

juice of 1 lemon

1 large handful of cilantro leaves, chopped

1 large handful of flat-leaf parsley leaves, chopped

sea salt

1   Preheat the oven to 350°F. Put the carrots and beets in a large roasting pan and the fennel, eggplants, and peppers in another large roasting pan. Drizzle half of the oil into the two pans and toss well to coat. First roast the carrots and beets 10 minutes, then put the other roasting pan in the oven and roast both 30 to 35 minutes longer, or until all the vegetables are slightly brown and tender.

2   Meanwhile, heat the remaining olive oil in a saucepan over medium heat. Add the onion and cook, stirring occasionally, 2 minutes. Add the quinoa and cook, stirring occasionally, 4 to 5 minutes longer until evenly brown. Add 2½ cups water and bring to a boil over high heat. Reduce the heat to low and simmer 20 minutes, or until tender, adding a little extra water, if necessary.

3   Mix the vegetables and quinoa together in a large bowl, then add the cumin, ground coriander, lemon juice, and cilantro and parsley leaves. Season with salt and serve either hot or cold.

lunches

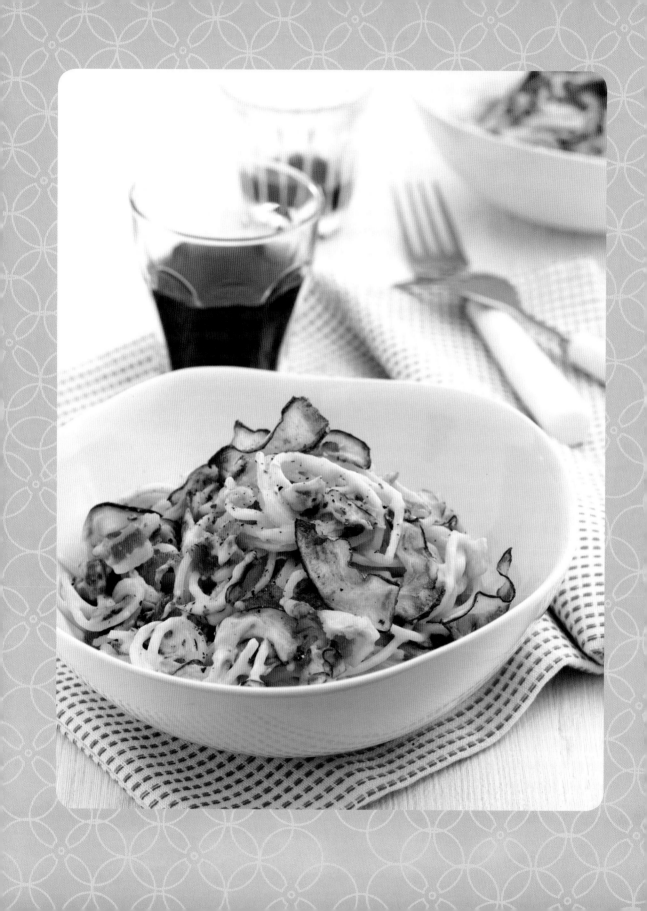

There's something truly wonderful about eating a good gluten- and dairy-free version of a classic recipe. Here I've added fried zucchini for toasted, sweet flavors and strongly aromatic sage to make a truly comforting meal.

Zucchini and Sage Spaghetti Carbonara

Serves **4**   Preparation time **15 minutes**   Cooking time **25 minutes**

½ cup olive oil

2 zucchini, trimmed, halved, and shaved into ribbons, using a vegetable peeler

14 ounces gluten-free spaghetti

10 ounces pancetta

1 heaped tablespoon chopped sage leaves

4 extra-large egg yolks

⅓ cup soy cream

2 cups grated soy cheese

sea salt and freshly ground black pepper

1   Heat 6 tablespoons of the oil in a wok or large skillet over medium heat. Working in batches, add a large handful of the zucchini ribbons and fry, stirring occasionally, 5 to 6 minutes until soft and light brown. With a slotted spoon, remove the zucchini from the pan and set aside.

2   Bring a large saucepan of water to a boil. Add 1 tablespoon of the remaining oil, then the spaghetti, pushing it down into the water as it softens. Cook over medium-high heat 8 to 10 minutes, or according to the package directions, stirring frequently to make sure the spaghetti doesn't stick together.

3   Meanwhile, heat the remaining tablespoon of the oil in a skillet over medium heat. Add the pancetta and fry, stirring occasionally, 5 to 6 minutes until crisp. Remove the pancetta from the pan with a slotted spoon and set aside. Add the sage and fry 1 to 2 minutes until crisp. Set aside, reserving the fat in the pan.

4   In a medium bowl, whisk together the egg yolks and soy cream, then whisk in the soy cheese and set aside.

5   Drain the spaghetti and rinse well with boiling water, then drain again briefly, leaving a little of the water remaining. Put the spaghetti back in the saucepan and quickly stir in the egg mixture. Quickly add the zucchini, pancetta, and sage, along with all of the fat remaining in the pan. Stir well and season with salt and pepper, then serve immediately.

I love baking—when I open the door of the oven and take out the finished result, it feels like I've created something wonderful. This tart is brimming with the beautiful tastes and fresh aromas of summertime.

Tomato Tart

Serves **4**   Preparation time **5 minutes, plus making the pastry**   Cooking time **50 minutes**

dairy-free margarine, for greasing

2 eggplants

1 recipe quantity Light Pastry Dough
   (see page 18)

brown rice flour, for dusting

6 tablespoons sun-dried tomato paste

6 or 7 tomatoes, sliced and end pieces discarded

12 cherry tomatoes, cut in half lengthwise

1 small handful of basil leaves, finely chopped

sea salt and freshly ground black pepper

1 Preheat the oven to 400°F and grease a loose-bottomed 12- x 8-inch tart pan with dairy-free margarine. Prick the eggplants all over with a fork, put them in a baking tray, and bake 45 minutes, or until very soft.

2 Meanwhile, liberally dust a large cutting board with rice flour and gently roll out the dough to about ¼ inch thick. Put the loose bottom of the tart pan on top of the dough and, using a sharp knife, cut around it. Shape the dough trimmings into a ball and set aside. Lift the cutting board and turn it over to drop the dough and bottom into the pan.

3 Dust the cutting board again with rice flour and gently roll out the remaining dough again. Cut it into strips wide enough to line the sides of the pan. To secure the sides of the tart, lightly brush some water along the bottom edges of the dough strips that will overlap with the bottom. Gently press the dough into the sides of the pan and along the bottom edge where it overlaps with the dough on the bottom, taking care to remove any air pockets. Neaten the edges, using a sharp knife, then prick the bottom of the dough with a fork. Line the tart case with a piece of baking parchment and fill with baking beans. Bake alongside the eggplants 15 minutes until light golden. Take the tart case out of the oven and remove the parchment and beans, then bake 2 to 3 minutes longer.

4 Remove the eggplants from the oven and turn the oven down to 350°F. Cut the eggplants in half and, using a spoon, scoop the flesh into a bowl. Mash well with a fork, then mix in the sun-dried tomato paste. Spread the eggplant and tomato mixture over the bottom of the tart shell and cover with the sliced tomatoes, followed by the cherry tomatoes.

5 Sprinkle with the basil and season with salt and pepper. Bake 20 to 25 minutes until the pastry is golden brown. Serve either hot or cold.

lunches

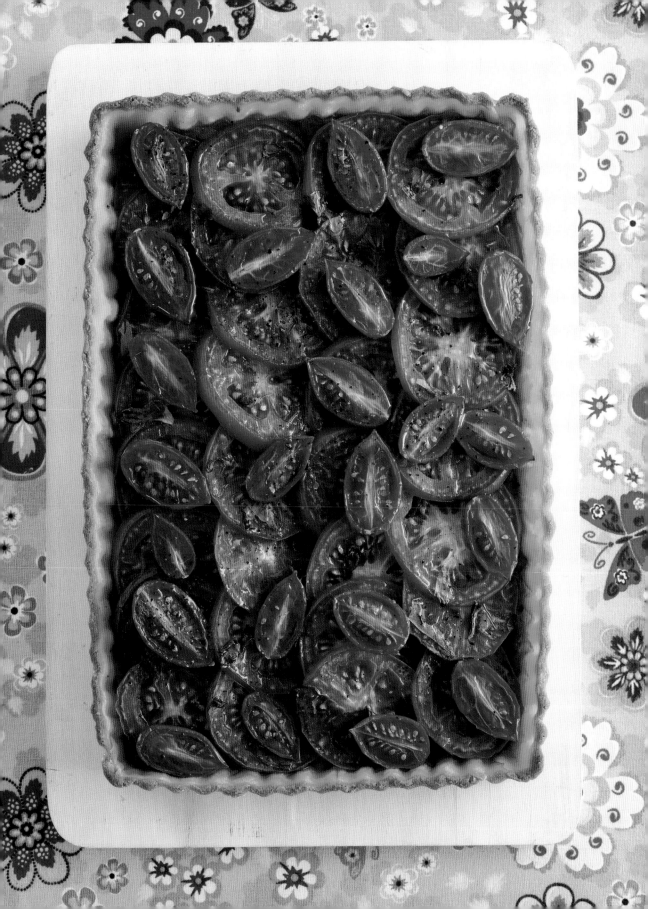

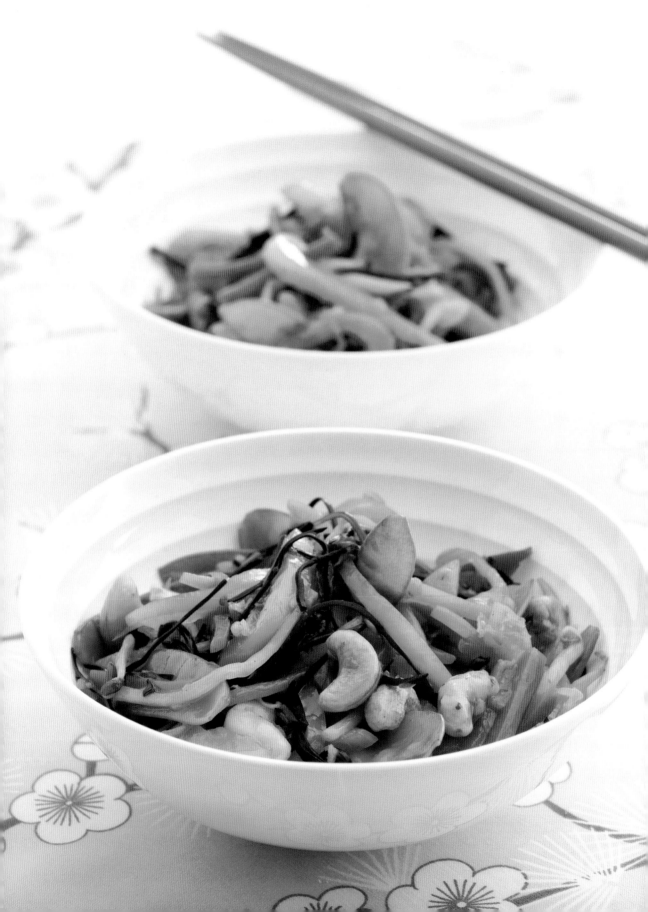

Arame is my favorite sea vegetable. It has a delicious, nutty taste and an exceptional nutritional profile, providing incredible quantities of calcium, iron, and magnesium, as well as phytonutrients.

Arame and Cashew Nut Stir-Fry

Serves **4**   Preparation time **15 minutes, plus 30 minutes soaking**   Cooking time **10 minutes**

¾ ounce arame

1 tablespoon kuzu

2 tablespoons toasted sesame oil

2 tablespoons olive oil

1 onion, finely chopped

2 garlic cloves, crushed

1-inch piece of ginger root, peeled and finely
   chopped

2 carrots, cut into matchsticks

2 yellow or orange bell peppers, seeded and
   finely sliced

1½ cups thinly sliced Chinese cabbage

5 ounces snow peas

2¼ cups bean sprouts

2½ tablespoons tamari soy sauce, plus extra,
   if needed

2½ tablespoons rice wine vinegar

2½ tablespoons agave syrup

½ cup Vegetable Stock (see page 21) or
   vegetable stock made from gluten- and
   dairy-free bouillon powder

1 cup cashew nuts

1   Soak the arame in a bowl of cold water about 30 minutes, then drain and rinse. Meanwhile, put the kuzu and 1 tablespoon cold water in a small bowl and stir to form a smooth paste, then set aside.

2   Heat both of the oils in a wok or large skillet over high heat. Add the onion and stir-fry 1 minute, then stir in the garlic and ginger. Add the carrot, pepper, and cabbage and stir-fry 2 to 3 minutes. Add the snow peas, bean sprouts, and drained arame and stir-fry 2 minutes longer.

3   Mix in the tamari, rice wine vinegar, and agave syrup, then add the kuzu paste and stock. Cook, stirring, 2 to 3 minutes longer until all of the vegetables are cooked but remain very crunchy.

4   Stir in the cashew nuts. Check the seasoning and add extra tamari if needed. Serve hot.

This collection of meze recipes makes a great lunch for friends and family, either in small or large numbers. Make everything the night before and enjoy a relaxing day!

Pomegranate Yogurt Dip

Serves **4**   Preparation time **10 minutes**   Cooking time **5 minutes**

⅓ cup pine nuts

1½ cups unflavored soy yogurt

2 pomegranates

1 garlic clove, crushed

1 handful of mint leaves, chopped

1 handful of cilantro leaves, chopped

sea salt

1   Heat a heavy-bottomed skillet over medium heat. Add the pine nuts and cook, stirring continuously, 3 to 4 minutes until just beginning to brown. Remove from the heat and set aside.

2   Whisk the yogurt in a large bowl until smooth. Halve the pomegranates and, holding each half over the bowl, bash the outer skin with a wooden spoon until all of the seeds fall into the bowl. You'll need to bash the skin a few times before the seeds begin to fall out, but they will. Add the pine nuts, garlic, and mint and cilantro leaves and mix well. Season lightly with salt and serve immediately or cover and keep in the refrigerator until needed.

Eggplant Spread

Serves **4**   Preparation time **10 minutes**   Cooking time **45 minutes**

2 eggplants

3 tablespoons tahini

juice of 2 lemons

2 garlic cloves, crushed

2 tablespoons olive oil

1 large handful of parsley leaves, chopped

1 handful of mint leaves, chopped

sea salt

1   Preheat the oven to 400°F. Prick the eggplants all over with a fork, put them in a baking tray, and bake 45 minutes, or until soft. Cut in half and, using a spoon, scoop the flesh into a food processor. Add the tahini, lemon juice, garlic, and oil. Season lightly with salt.

2   Blend well, then transfer to a bowl and stir in the parsley and mint. Serve immediately, or cover and keep in the refrigerator until needed.

Fennel and Tomato Salad

Serves **4**   Preparation time **15 minutes**

2 fennel bulbs

½ cucumber, diced

½ red onion, sliced

4 tomatoes, diced

juice of 1 lemon

¼ cup olive oil

1 large handful of cilantro leaves, chopped

1 large handful of parsley leaves, chopped

sea salt

1   Trim off the leafy fronds at the top of the fennel and put them in a salad bowl. Slice the fennel bulbs in half lengthwise, then slice thinly and add to the bowl. Add all of the remaining ingredients and stir well.

2   Season lightly with salt and serve immediately, or cover and keep in the refrigerator until needed.

Cannellini Bean Dip

Serves **4**   Preparation time **10 minutes, plus at least 12 hours soaking (optional)**
Cooking time **1 hour 40 minutes**

½ cup dried cannellini beans or 1¼ cups
   drained canned cannellini beans, rinsed

a pinch of ground cumin

1 garlic clove, crushed

1 tablespoon pomegranate molasses

1 tablespoon lemon juice

scant ½ teaspoon harissa paste

3 tablespoons olive oil

sea salt

1   If using dried cannellini beans, put them in a bowl, cover with cold water, and let soak overnight, or for at least 12 hours, then drain and rinse well. Transfer to a large saucepan, cover with fresh water, and bring to a boil over high heat. Boil 10 minutes, then turn the heat down to medium and simmer, covered, 1 to 1½ hours until tender. Drain well.

2   Put all of the ingredients in a food processor, season with salt, and blend 3 to 4 minutes until smooth. Let cool, then serve or cover and keep in the refrigerator until needed.

Baked Treats

Baking can be ridiculously easy — and wonderfully satisfying.
The aromas that envelop the kitchen and the creations that
come out of the oven seem almost magical. And perhaps even more
so when you're cooking without gluten or dairy. Turn the oven on, line
up the ingredients, and start mixing — it's good for the soul! Dive into
rich Chocolate and Mango Florentines, sweet Apricot, Yogurt, and
Honey Cake, or light, fluffy Almond Cake, for example. Add another
bread to your repertoire with delicious Fruit Loaf; make a little piece
of heaven with Raspberry and Rosewater Cupcakes or Portuguese
Custard Tarts; or whip up a stunning Chocolate Birthday Cake.

Apple Cake, page 100 >

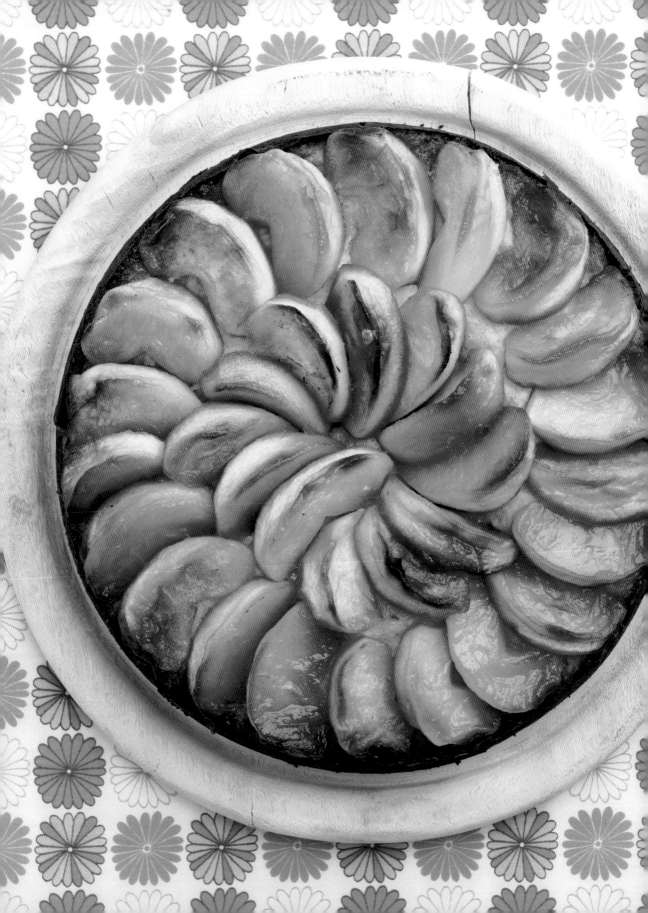

I've used figs to add moisture to these delicious cookies, hold them together, and add a crunchy chewiness — but also because they make them a seriously healthy version of a chocolate cookie!

Chocolate and Fig Cookies

Makes **12**   Preparation time **15 minutes**   Cooking time **40 minutes**

1 cup dried figs, stems discarded, finely chopped

6 tablespoons plus 2 teaspoons dairy-free margarine

½ cup fruit sugar or granulated sugar

3½ ounces dairy-free dark chocolate, 70% cocoa solids, broken into small pieces

1 egg, beaten

2 teaspoons vanilla extract

⅔ cup brown rice flour

heaped ½ cup chickpea flour

scant ½ cup corn flour

½ teaspoon gluten-free baking powder

½ teaspoon xanthan gum

1 Preheat the oven to 350°F and line two cookie sheets with baking parchment. Put the figs and 1½ cups water in a saucepan, bring to a boil over high heat, then turn the heat down to medium. Simmer 20 minutes, stirring occasionally, until the figs soften and the water is absorbed.

2 Meanwhile, put the dairy-free margarine and sugar in a saucepan and heat over low heat until the dairy-free margarine melts and the sugar dissolves. Bring to a boil over high heat, then turn the heat down to medium-low and simmer 4 to 5 minutes until the mixture becomes syrupy and slightly darker in color.

3 When the sugar mixture changes color, turn the heat to low and add the chocolate. Continue simmering, stirring occasionally, until it melts. Add the egg and vanilla extract and mix well. Pour the mixture into a large mixing bowl and sift in the flours, gluten-free baking powder, and xanthan gum. Add the softened figs and stir well until mixed.

4 Shape 1 tablespoon of the dough into a ball with your hands and place on the cookie sheet, pressing the tines of a fork gently over the surface to score lightly. Repeat with the remaining dough to make 12 cookies.

5 Bake 20 minutes, or until lightly browned. Remove from the oven and let cool 5 minutes, then transfer to a wire rack and let cool completely before serving.

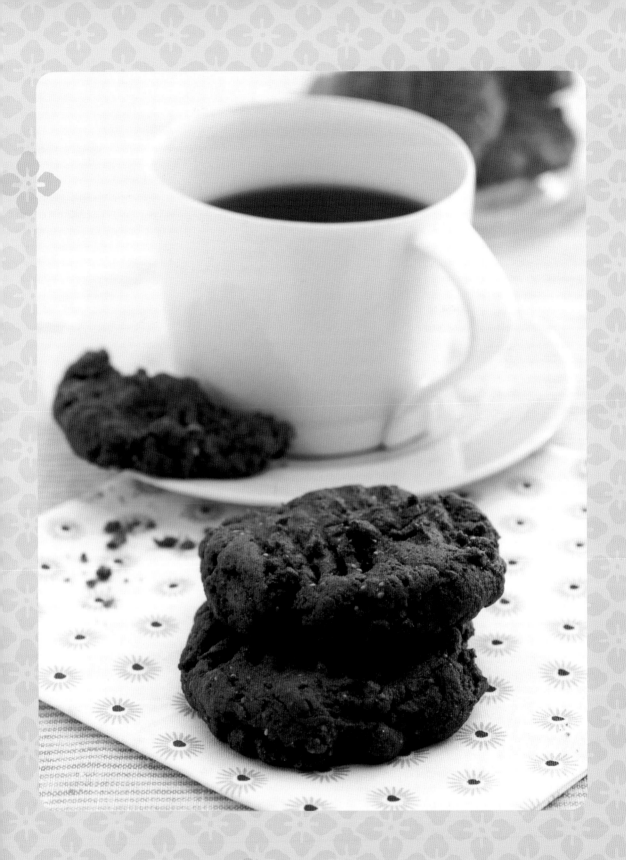

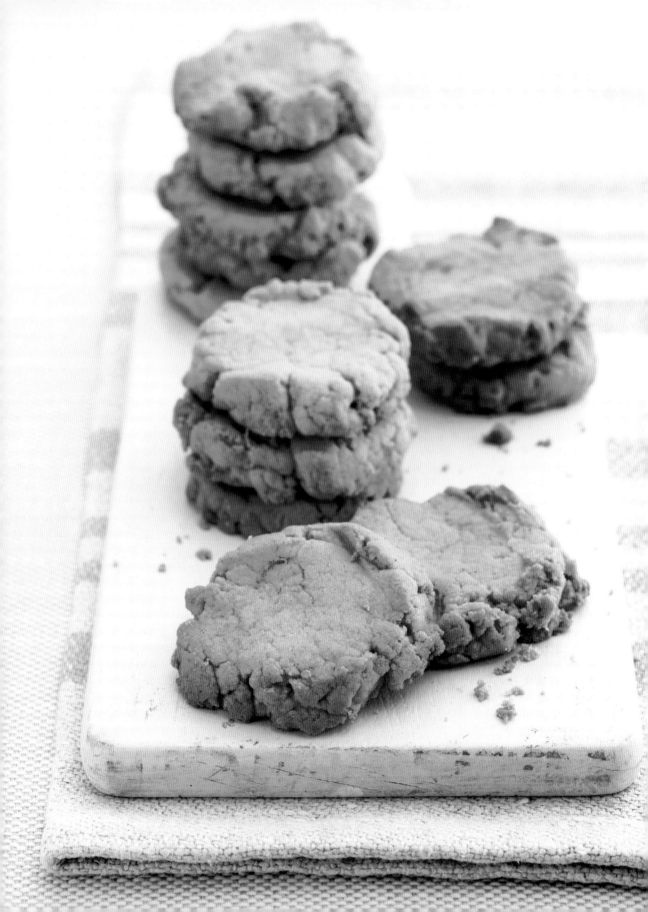

These cookies were one of the things I loved eating when I was pregnant and suffering from morning sickness. They're very simple to make—and the ginger in them soothes digestive problems and eases nausea.

Ginger Cookies

Makes **12**   Preparation time **15 minutes**   Cooking time **20 minutes**

¾ cup dairy-free margarine

1 cup plus 2 tablespoons fruit sugar
  or granulated sugar

⅔ cup brown rice flour

heaped ½ cup chickpea flour

scant ½ cup corn flour

2 teaspoons ground ginger

½ teaspoon gluten-free baking powder

scant ½ teaspoon xanthan gum

½-inch piece of ginger root, peeled and grated

1   Preheat the oven to 350°F and line two cookie sheets with baking parchment. Put the dairy-free margarine and sugar in a saucepan and heat over low heat until the margarine melts and the sugar dissolves. Bring to a boil over high heat, then turn the heat down to medium-low and simmer 4 to 5 minutes until the mixture caramelizes slightly and becomes syrupy.

2   Sift the flours into a large mixing bowl and stir in the ground ginger, gluten-free baking powder, and xanthan gum. Add the ginger root and, using your fingertips, rub it into the flour mixture until well mixed. Add the margarine and sugar syrup, and stir well.

3   Spoon the cookie dough, 1 tablespoon at a time, onto the cookie sheets. Using your hands and the back of a metal spoon, shape each mound into a round cookie shape about ⅛ inch thick.

4   Bake 8 to 12 minutes until light brown. Remove the cookie sheets from the oven and let the cookies to cool 5 minutes, then transfer to a wire rack and let cool completely before serving.

baked treats

This is a healthy twist on the classic Florentine recipe, using dried mango instead of sugar-loaded candied peel and cherries.

Mango and Hazelnut Florentines

Makes **8 to 10**   Preparation time **15 minutes, plus 30 minutes chilling**   Cooking time **35 minutes**

3½ ounces dried mango, chopped

5 tablespoons dairy-free margarine, plus extra
    for greasing

scant ½ cup fruit sugar or granulated sugar

1 tablespoon brown rice flour

1 tablespoon chickpea flour

1 tablespoon corn flour

¼ teaspoon xanthan gum

⅓ cup chopped hazelnuts

3½ ounces dairy-free dark chocolate,
    70% cocoa solids, chopped

1 Preheat the oven to 350°F. Line two cookie sheets with baking parchment and grease them with dairy-free margarine. Put the dried mango and 1 cup plus 2 tablespoons water in a saucepan. Bring to a boil over high heat, then turn the heat down to medium and simmer 15 to 20 minutes until the mango softens and the water is absorbed.

2 Meanwhile, put the dairy-free margarine and sugar in a saucepan and heat over low heat until the margarine melts and the sugar dissolves. Bring to a boil over high heat, then turn the heat down to medium-low and simmer 4 to 5 minutes until the mixture has caramelizes slightly and become syrupy.

3 Sift the flours and xanthan gum into a large mixing bowl. Add the hazelnuts, softened mango, and margarine and sugar syrup. Stir well with a wooden spoon until mixed. Spoon the dough, 1 tablespoon at a time, onto the cookie sheets to make 8 to 10 balls, leaving some space between each one. Press down on each mound with the back of the spoon to make a round cookie shape, about 1⁄16in thick. Bake 10 to 12 minutes until light brown. Remove the cookie sheets from the oven and leave the cookies to cool 5 minutes, then transfer to a wire rack and leave to cool completely.

4 Meanwhile, put the chocolate in a large heatproof bowl and rest it over a pan of gently simmering water, making sure he bottom of the bowl does not touch the water. Stir occasionally until the chocolate melts. When the cookies are cool, put them flat-side up on a plate and carefully spoon some of the melted chocolate on top of each one and spread it over evenly. Chill the cookies in the refrigerator 30 minutes, or until the chocolate sets, then serve.

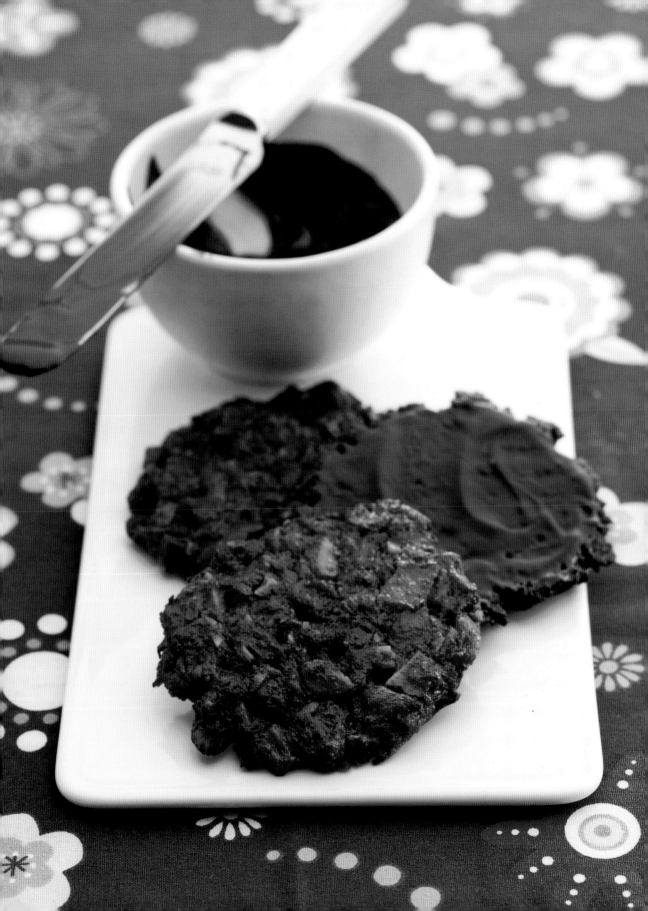

Hemp seeds, figs, dates, and pomegranate molasses provide a Moroccan twist to this gooey yet crunchy fruit-and-nut bar.

Fig and Date Fruit Bars

Makes **8**   Preparation time **15 minutes**   Cooking time **35 minutes**

dairy-free margarine, for greasing

1⅓ cups dried figs, stems discarded, chopped

¾ cup chopped pitted dates

⅓ cup pine nuts

1 tablespoon pomegranate molasses

2 tablespoons agave syrup

heaped 1 cup rice flakes

1 tablespoon hemp seeds

1   Preheat the oven to 350°F. Grease two 8½- x 4½-inch bread pans with dairy-free margarine and line the bottom with baking parchment. Put the figs, dates, and 1½ cups plus 2 tablespoons water in a saucepan and bring to a boil over high heat, then turn the heat down to medium and simmer 15 minutes, or until the fruit softens and the water is absorbed.

2   Meanwhile, heat a heavy-bottomed skillet over medium heat until hot. Add the pine nuts and heat, stirring frequently, until light brown, then transfer to a large mixing bowl.

3   Add the softened fruit, pomegranate molasses, and agave syrup to the bowl and mix well. Add the rice flakes and stir well, using a wooden spoon. Divide the mixture evenly between the two bread pans and level the surfaces with the back of a spoon. Sprinkle the hemp seeds over the tops and press down firmly with your fingertips.

4   Bake 18 to 20 minutes until lightly browned and firm. Remove from the oven and let cool in the pans 5 minutes, then cut each one into 4 bars. Gently ease them out of the pans and let cool completely on a wire rack before serving.

baked treats

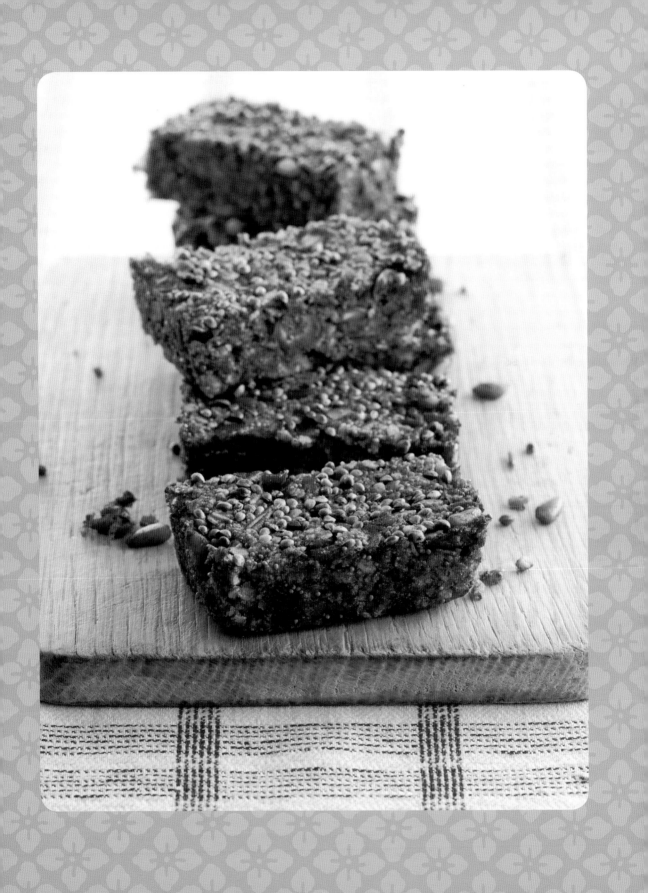

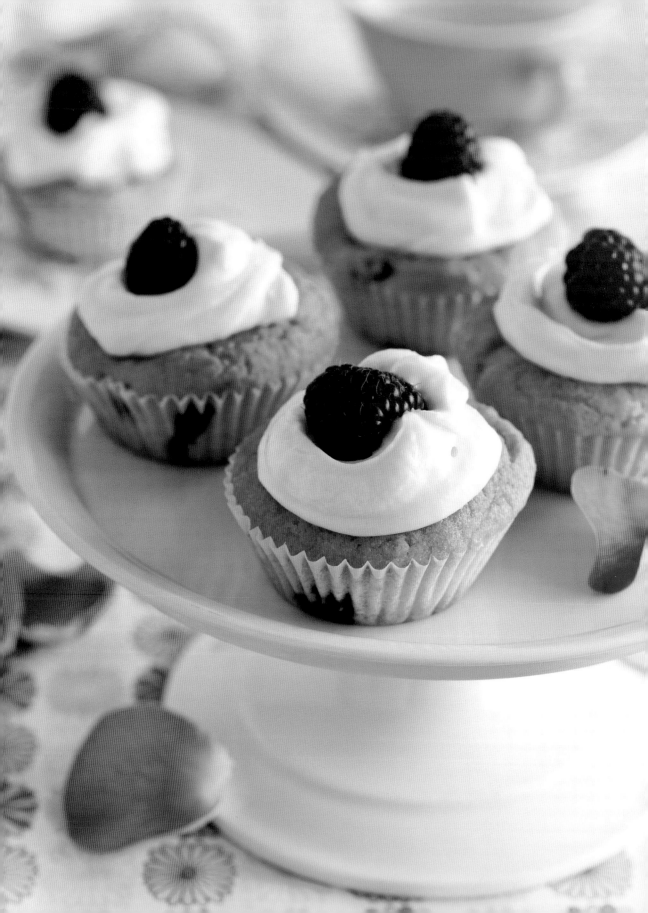

Ground almonds make these cupcakes deliciously light and moist. Covered with a thick, silky rosewater-flavored frosting, they are truly indulgent!

Raspberry and Rosewater Cupcakes

Makes 12   Preparation time **15 minutes**   Cooking time **25 minutes**

⅔ cup dairy-free margarine, softened

½ cup plus 2 tablespoons fruit sugar or
   granulated sugar

3 large eggs

heaped ½ cup brown rice flour

1 teaspoon gluten-free baking powder

scant ½ teaspoon xanthan gum

¾ cup very finely ground blanched almonds

scant 1 cup raspberries, lightly mashed,
   plus 12 to decorate

ROSEWATER FROSTING:

2 tablespoons dairy-free margarine

5 tablespoons soy cream cheese

1 teaspoon rosewater

½ cup less 1 tablespoon fruit sugar
   or granulated sugar

1 Preheat the oven to 350°F and arrange 12 paper cupcake cases in a muffin pan. To make the frosting, put the dairy-free margarine, soy cream cheese, and rosewater in a mixing bowl and beat, using a whisk or an electric mixer, until smooth. Add the sugar, a little at a time, and beat until light and fluffy. Cover and chill in the refrigerator 30 minutes.

2 Using an electric mixer, beat the dairy-free margarine and sugar together in a large mixing bowl until light and fluffy. Gradually beat in the eggs, one at a time, until well mixed.

3 Sift the rice flour, gluten-free baking powder, and xanthan gum into the mixture. Quickly fold in the ground almonds, using a spoon, then gently fold in the raspberries. Mix well, but take care not to overmix. Divide the batter evenly into the cupcake cases.

4 Bake 18 to 20 minutes until golden brown, well risen, and a skewer inserted in the middle comes out clean. Remove the muffin pan from the oven and turn the cupcake out of the pan, then transfer to a wire rack and let cool completely.

5 Spread a little of the frosting over each cupcake, top with a raspberry, and serve.

baked treats

Nutmeg is naturally sweet and, when combined with vanilla extract, it creates a rich, warm flavor for the light, creamy filling in these tarts.

Portuguese Custard Tarts

Makes **4**   Preparation time **15 minutes, plus making the dough**   Cooking time **35 minutes**

dairy-free margarine, for greasing

brown rice flour, for dusting

1 recipe quantity Sweet Piecrust Dough with
    ½ teaspoon freshly grated nutmeg added
    (see page 19)

1¾ cups soy milk

1½ tablespoons cornstarch

½ cup less 1 tablespoon fruit sugar or
    granulated sugar

scant 1 teaspoon vanilla extract

1 teaspoon freshly grated nutmeg, plus extra
    for sprinkling

4 extra-large egg yolks, beaten

1   Preheat the oven to 400°F and grease four 4-inch loose-bottomed tartlet pans with dairy-free margarine. Liberally dust a work surface with rice flour and gently roll out the dough to about ⅛ inch thick. Be very gentle, as the dough will still be slightly sticky. Using a cookie cutter that is slightly larger in diameter than the tartlet pans (to allow enough dough for the sides), cut out four circles. Gather up the dough trimmings, wrap in plastic wrap, and freeze for use another time.

2   Lift the pastry circles into each pan (you might need to use a metal spatula) and press down lightly to remove any air pockets. Neaten the edges, using a sharp knife, then line each tart shell with a piece of baking parchment, cover with baking beans, and put them on a baking sheet. Bake 8 to 10 minutes until firm and very lightly golden. Remove from the oven and turn the oven down to 350°F.

3   Meanwhile, heat the soy milk in a heavy-bottomed saucepan over low heat until almost boiling. While the soy milk is warming, mix together the cornstarch and 1 tablespoon water in a small bowl and stir until smooth. Whisk the paste, sugar, vanilla extract, and nutmeg into the hot milk, then whisk in the egg yolks a little bit at a time until incorporated. Cook over low heat, stirring frequently, 10 to 15 minutes until a thick custard forms. Be careful not to overheat or it can curdle; if it does, beat with a whisk until smooth.

4   Remove the baking parchment and beans and fill the tart shells with the custard, using a small ladle. Sprinkle a little nutmeg over the tarts and bake 15 minutes, or until set. Remove from the oven and leave the tarts to cool 5 minutes. Lift them out of the pans and either serve warm or transfer to a wire rack to cool before serving. Chill any leftover tarts.

baked treats

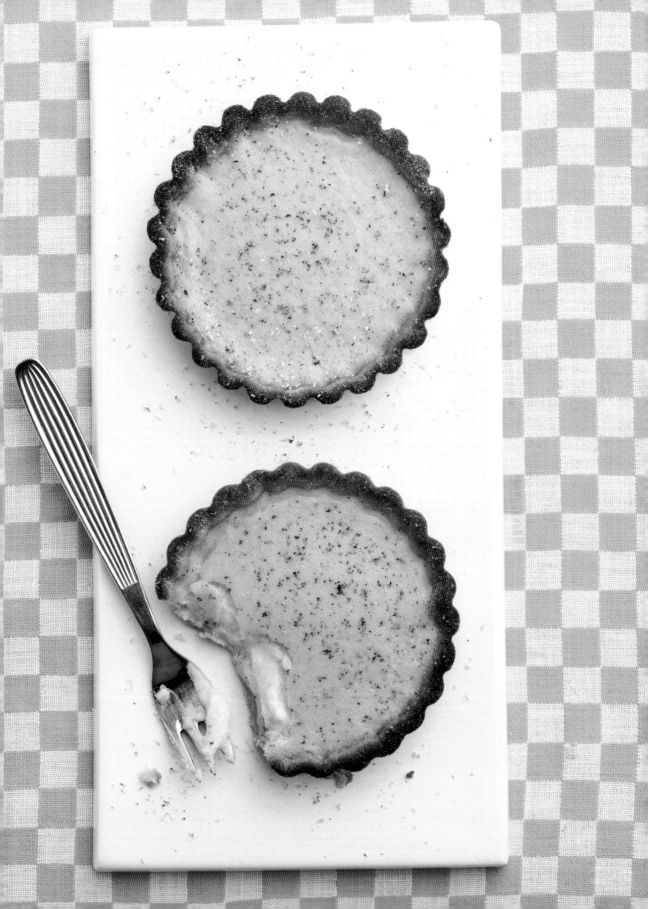

Soya yogurt has a delicious, tangy taste and a smooth, creamy texture when blended. Here it adds moisture and velvety thickness to the cake batter — and makes a cool, light topping.

Apricot, Yogurt, and Honey Cake

Makes **1 cake (10 to 12 slices)**   Preparation time **15 minutes**   Cooking time **50 minutes**

⅔ cup dairy-free margarine, softened, plus extra
   for greasing

1 cup plus 2 tablespoons fruit sugar or
   granulated sugar

2 large eggs, beaten

1 teaspoon vanilla extract

¼ cup honey

1 cup plus 2 tablespoons unflavored soy yogurt

⅔ cup brown rice flour

heaped ½ cup chickpea flour

scant ½ cup corn flour

2 teaspoon gluten-free baking powder

½ teaspoon xanthan gum

heaped 1 cup unsulfured dried apricots,
   finely chopped

TOPPING:

6 tablespoons unflavored soy yogurt

2 tablespoons honey

1   Preheat the oven to 350°F and lightly grease a deep 8-inch cake pan with dairy-free margarine and line the bottom with baking parchment. Using an electric mixer, beat the dairy-free margarine and sugar together in a large mixing bowl until light and fluffy. Gradually beat in the eggs, a little at a time, until well mixed, then beat in the vanilla extract, honey, and soy yogurt.

2   Sift the flours, gluten-free baking powder, and xanthan gum into the mixture and fold in, then fold in the chopped apricots. Make sure the mixture is well mixed, but take care not to overmix it. Pour it into the pan.

3   Bake 30 minutes, then cover with baking parchment to prevent the cake overbrowning. Bake 15 to 20 minutes longer until firm to the touch and baked through.

4   Meanwhile, prepare the topping. Using a whisk or electric mixer, whisk the yogurt and honey together in a bowl until smooth. Keep cool in the refrigerator until needed.

5   Remove the cake from the oven and let cool 5 minutes, then remove from the pan, transfer to a wire rack and let cool completely. Once cool, spread the topping over the cake and serve. Store any leftover cake in the refrigerator.

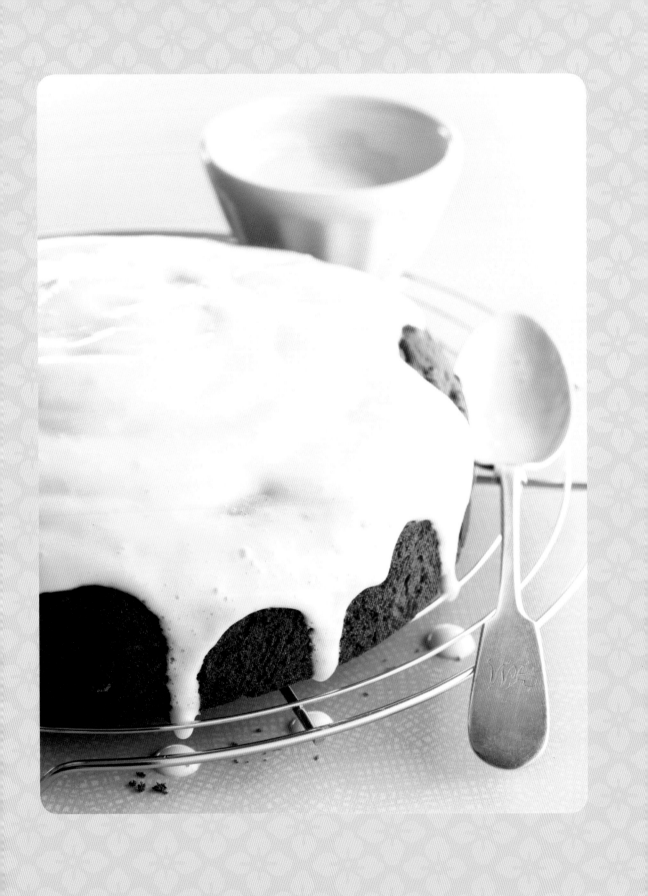

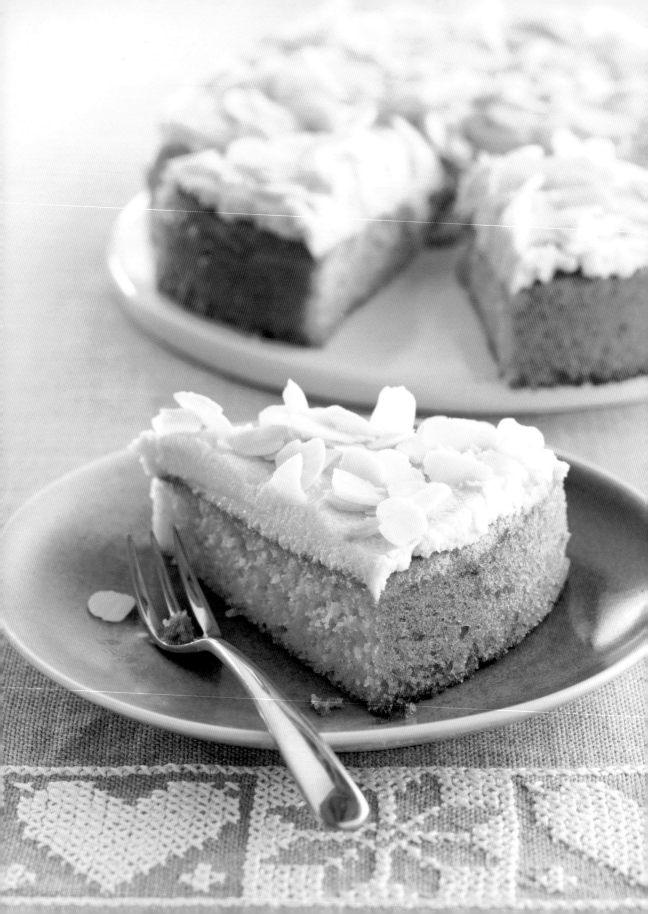

Thanks to the ground almonds, this cake comes out of the oven light, fluffy, and moist. The flavors are delicate, and the almond cream and flaked almonds add a rich coating with a crunchy top.

Almond Cake

Makes **1 cake (10 to 12 slices)**   Preparation time **20 minutes, plus at least 12 hours soaking**
Cooking time **35 minutes**

⅔ cup dairy-free margarine, softened, plus extra
    for greasing
6 tablespoons fruit sugar or granulated sugar
1 teaspoon almond extract
3 large eggs, beaten
heaped 1 cup finely ground blanched almonds
1 teaspoon gluten-free baking powder
scant ½ teaspoon xanthan gum
⅓ cup slivered almonds, to decorate

ALMOND CREAM:
⅔ cup blanched almonds
2 tablespoons fruit sugar or granulated sugar
¼ teaspoon almond extract
2 teaspoons agar agar flakes

1   To make the almond cream, put the blanched almonds in a bowl, cover with water, and let
    soak overnight, or for at least 12 hours, then drain, rinse well, and transfer to a blender. Add
    ⅔ cup water and blend 10 minutes until smooth. Pour the mixture into a saucepan and
    add the sugar, almond extract, and agar agar flakes. Heat over low heat 3 to 4 minutes until
    the sugar and agar agar flakes dissolve completely, stirring continuously to make sure the
    mixture doesn't burn. Transfer to a heatproof bowl, let cool, then cover and chill in
    the refrigerator until needed.

2   Preheat the oven to 350°F and lightly grease an 8-inch cake pan with dairy-free margarine
    and line the bottom with baking parchment. Using an electric mixer, beat the dairy-free
    margarine and sugar together in a large mixing bowl until light and fluffy. Beat in the almond
    extract and gradually beat in the eggs, a little at a time, until well mixed. Add the ground
    almonds, gluten-free baking powder, and xanthan gum to the mixture, then quickly fold
    in, using a large spoon. Mix well, but take care not to overmix, then pour into the pan.

3   Bake 20 to 25 minutes until golden brown, well risen, and a skewer inserted in the middle
    comes out clean. Remove from the oven and let cool 5 minutes. Turn out of the pan, transfer
    to a wire rack, and let cool completely.

4   Spread the almond cream over the cake, sprinkle with the slivered almonds, and serve.
    Keep any leftover cake in the refrigerator.

baked treats

I've used quinoa flour in this cake and a mixture of rice flour and ground almonds. The almonds and dried fruits sweeten and enrich the quinoa's distinctive, nutty taste.

Fruit Cake

Makes **1 cake (12 to 14 slices)**   Preparation time **20 minutes**   Cooking time **1 hour 25 minutes**

1 cup dairy-free margarine, plus extra for
  greasing

1⅓ cups raisins

1⅓ cups golden raisins

scant 2 cups unsulfured dried apricots, chopped

¼ cup dried sour cherries

⅓ cup dried cranberries

2 tablespoons dried goji berries

scant 1 cup blanched hazelnuts

⅔ cup brown rice flour

heaped 1 cup quinoa flour

⅔ cup very finely ground blanched almonds

¼ teaspoon salt

2 teaspoons cinnamon

1½ teaspoons gluten-free baking powder

heaped ½ teaspoon xanthan gum

1 cup fruit sugar or granulated sugar

4 extra-large eggs, beaten

1   Preheat the oven to 350°F and lightly grease a 9-inch springform cake pan with dairy-free margarine. Put the raisins, golden raisins, apricots, cherries, cranberries, goji berries, and 4½ cups less 2 tablespoons water in a saucepan. Bring to a boil over high heat, then turn the heat down to medium and simmer 30 to 40 minutes until all of the fruit softens and the water is absorbed.

2   Put the hazelnuts in a mini food processor and pulse until chopped.

3   Sift the flours, salt, cinnamon, gluten-free baking powder, and xanthan gum into a large mixing bowl. Add the ground almonds and mix well.

4   Using an electric mixer, beat the dairy-free margarine and sugar together in a large mixing bowl until light and fluffy. Gradually beat in the eggs, one at a time, until well mixed, then stir in the softened fruits and chopped hazelnuts, using a large spoon. Quickly fold in the flour mixture. Make sure the batter is well blended, but take care not to overmix. Pour the batter into the pan and smooth the surface with the back of a metal spoon.

5   Bake 30 minutes, then cover with baking parchment, tucking the ends under the pan securely. Bake 10 to 15 minutes longer until baked through. The cake will seem very gooey when it comes out of the oven, but it will set as it cools. Let cool in the pan 5 minutes, then turn it out and transfer to a wire rack. Let cool completely before serving.

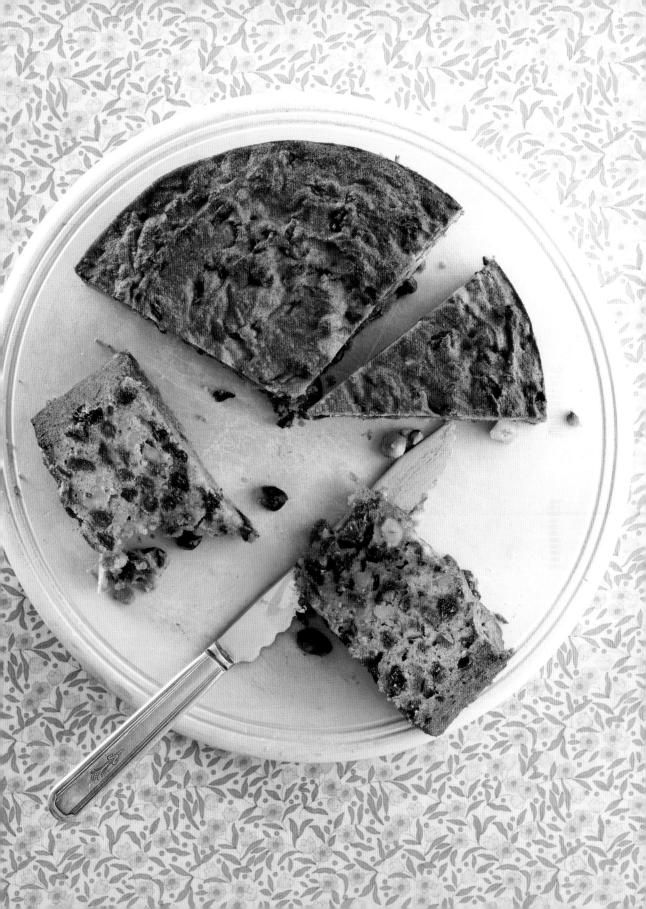

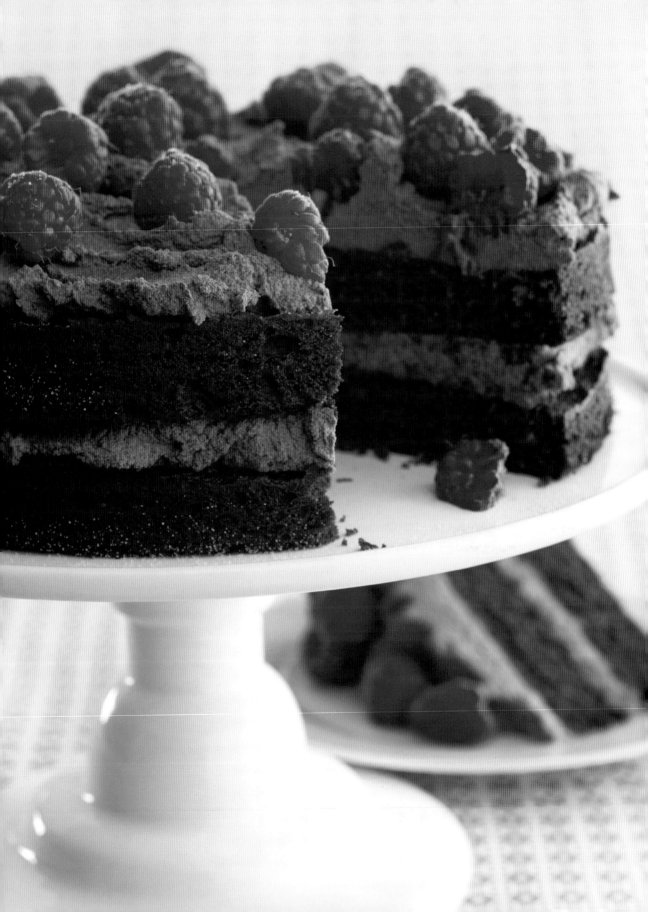

This heavenly cake was inspired by one my sister made for her husband's birthday. It's light and moist, with dark truffley chocolate flavors and a rich, creamy frosting, all covered with sweetly sharp raspberries.

Chocolate Birthday Cake

Makes **1 cake**   Preparation time **25 minutes, plus making the nut cream**   Cooking time **45 minutes**

⅔ cup dairy-free margarine, softened, plus extra
    for greasing

7 ounces dairy-free dark chocolate, 70% cocoa
    solids, chopped or broken into pieces

1 cup less 2 tablespoons fruit sugar or
    granulated sugar

1 teaspoon vanilla extract

4 extra-large eggs

heaped ⅓ cup brown rice flour

scant ⅓ cup chestnut flour

2 teaspoons gluten-free baking powder

½ teaspoon xanthan gum

1¼ cups raspberries, to decorate

FROSTING:

7 ounces dairy-free dark chocolate, 70% cocoa
    solids, chopped or broken into pieces

1 recipe quantity Cashew Nut Cream
    (see page 13), adding 1 teaspoon vanilla
    extract and 8 dates when blending

1   Preheat the oven to 350°F and lightly grease two 9-inch springform cake tins with dairy-free margarine. Put the chocolate in a large heatproof bowl and rest it over a pan of gently simmering water, making sure that the bottom of the bowl does not touch the water. Heat, stirring occasionally, until the chocolate melts.

2   Using an electric mixer, beat the dairy-free margarine and sugar together in a large mixing bowl until light and fluffy. Beat in the vanilla extract, then beat in the eggs, one at a time. Using a large spoon, carefully fold in the melted chocolate mixture. Sift the flours, gluten-free baking powder, and xanthan gum into the mixture and fold in, using a large spoon. Make sure the batter is well mixed, but take care not to overmix. Evenly divide the batter into the cake pans and level the surfaces. Bake 35 to 40 minutes until firm to the touch and a skewer inserted in the middle comes out clean. Remove from the oven and let cool in the pans 5 minutes, then turn out onto wire racks and let cool completely.

3   Meanwhile, put the chocolate for the frosting in a large heatproof bowl and follow the same procedure as in step 1, above, to melt. Put the blended nut cream and date mixture in a food processor or blender, add the melted chocolate, and blend until well mixed.

4   Put one of the cakes on a plate and spread half of the frosting over the top. Put the other cake on top, flat-side down, and spread the remaining frosting over the top. Decorate with the raspberries, then serve.

baked treats

This recipe is my homage to Dorset, in southern England, where I grew up. The sweet flavors and soft texture of the apples combine beautifully with the firm cake base.

Apple Cake

Makes **1 cake (10 to 12 slices)**   Preparation time **20 minutes**   Cooking time **50 minutes**

⅔ cup dairy-free margarine, softened, plus extra
    for greasing

4 apples, peeled, cored, and cut into large
    chunks

¼ cup agave syrup

½ cup plus 2 tablespoons fruit sugar
    or granulated sugar

1 teaspoon vanilla extract

3 extra-large eggs

⅔ cup brown rice flour

heaped ½ cup chickpea flour

1 teaspoon gluten-free baking powder

½ teaspoon xanthan gum

⅓ cup very finely ground blanched almonds

1 Preheat the oven to 350°F. Lightly grease a deep 8-inch cake pan with dairy-free margarine and line the bottom with baking parchment. Heat 1 tablespoon of the dairy-free margarine in a heavy-bottomed saucepan over low heat, then add the apples and cook 5 minutes, or until they are starting to brown, shaking the pan or gently stirring occasionally so they do not burn. Add the agave syrup and cook 5 minutes longer until soft, shaking the pan, occasionally, then set aside.

2 Meanwhile, using an electric mixer, beat the sugar and remaining dairy-free margarine together in a large mixing bowl until light and fluffy. Add the vanilla extract, then gradually beat in the eggs, one at a time, until well mixed.

3 Sift the flours, gluten-free baking powder, and xanthan gum into the mixture. Add the ground almonds and fold together, using a large spoon. Make sure the batter is well mixed, but take care not to overmix. Pour it into the pan and level the surface, using a clean knife. Arrange the apples on top (use the back of a spoon to even them, if needed) and pour the syrup from the pan evenly over the top. Bake 40 minutes, or until firm to the touch and baked through.

4 Remove the pan from the oven and leave the cake to cool 5 minutes, then turn out of the pan and transfer to a wire rack. Let cool completely before serving.

baked treats

Unlike most gluten-free flours, chestnut flour has great binding properties, so it's a wonderful choice for baking. Its distinctive taste can sometimes overpower others, but the two kinds of raisins used here complement it.

Fruit Loaf

Makes **1 loaf (about 16 slices)**   Preparation time **20 minutes, plus 30 minutes rising**
Cooking time **1 hour 10 minutes**

⅔ cup golden raisins

⅔ cup raisins

¾ cup potato flour

¾ cup brown rice flour

scant 1 cup chestnut flour

½ teaspoon fine sea salt

2 tablespoons fruit sugar or granulated sugar

1 teaspoon gluten-free baking powder

1 teaspoon xanthan gum

1 tablespoon active dry yeast

3 tablespoons plus 1 teaspoon dairy-free
    margarine, cut into cubes, plus extra
    for greasing

1   Put the golden raisins, raisins, and 1 cup plus 2 tablespoons water in a saucepan. Bring to a boil over high heat, then turn the heat down to medium and simmer 15 to 20 minutes until the fruit softens and the water is absorbed.

2   Sift the flours, salt, sugar, gluten-free baking powder, xanthan gum, and yeast into a food processor with the dough blade attached and blend to mix together. Add the dairy-free margarine and blend again, then add 1¾ cups warm water and process 10 minutes to aerate the dough. Add the softened golden raisins and raisins and mix well. Transfer the dough to a bowl, cover with plastic wrap, and let rise 30 minutes.

3   Preheat the oven to 400°F and lightly grease an 8½- x 4½-inch bread pan with dairy-free margarine. Spoon the dough into the pan and level the surface with the back of a spoon.

4   Bake 20 minutes, then brush some water over the top with a pastry brush and cover with baking parchment, tucking the ends under the pan securely. Bake 20 minutes longer, brush again with water, and then re-cover. Bake 5 to 10 minutes longer until baked through. Turn the cake out of the pan, transfer to a wire rack and let cool at least 10 minutes before serving.

baked treats

Packed with beta-carotene, butternut squash gives these scones moistness and texture. These are delicious with jam, fruit spread, or a savory spread.

Butternut Squash Scones

Makes **6**   Preparation time **25 minutes**   Cooking time **40 minutes**

scant 1 cup peeled, seeded, and chopped
  butternut squash

3 tablespoons plus 1 teaspoon dairy-free
  margarine, plus extra for greasing and
  to serve

heaped ½ cup brown rice flour, plus extra
  for dusting

heaped ⅓ cup corn flour

scant ⅓ cup chickpea flour

½ teaspoon xanthan gum

2 teaspoons gluten-free baking powder

a pinch of salt

2 tablespoons fruit sugar or granulated sugar

1 tablespoon unsweetened soy milk

jam, fruit spread, or savory spread, to serve

1   Put the squash in a steamer and steam over medium-high heat 15 minutes, or until soft.

2   Preheat the oven to 350°F and grease a baking sheet with dairy-free margarine. Sift the flours, xanthan gum, gluten-free baking powder, salt, and sugar into a food processor with the dough blade attached and blend 1 minute to mix well. Add the dairy-free margarine and blend 2 minutes to mix, then add the soy milk and scant ½ cup cooked squash and blend 10 minutes longer. The dough will be very sticky.

3   Dust a cutting board liberally with rice flour. Scoop the dough onto the board and lightly roll it in the rice flour until workable. With the palm of your hand, press the dough out evenly to about ¾ inch thick. Using a 2½-inch round cookie cutter, cut out the scones, reworking the dough as needed.

4   Put the scones on the baking sheet and bake 20 to 25 minutes until golden brown. Serve warm with dairy-free margarine and jam, or turn out onto a wire rack to cool before serving.

baked treats

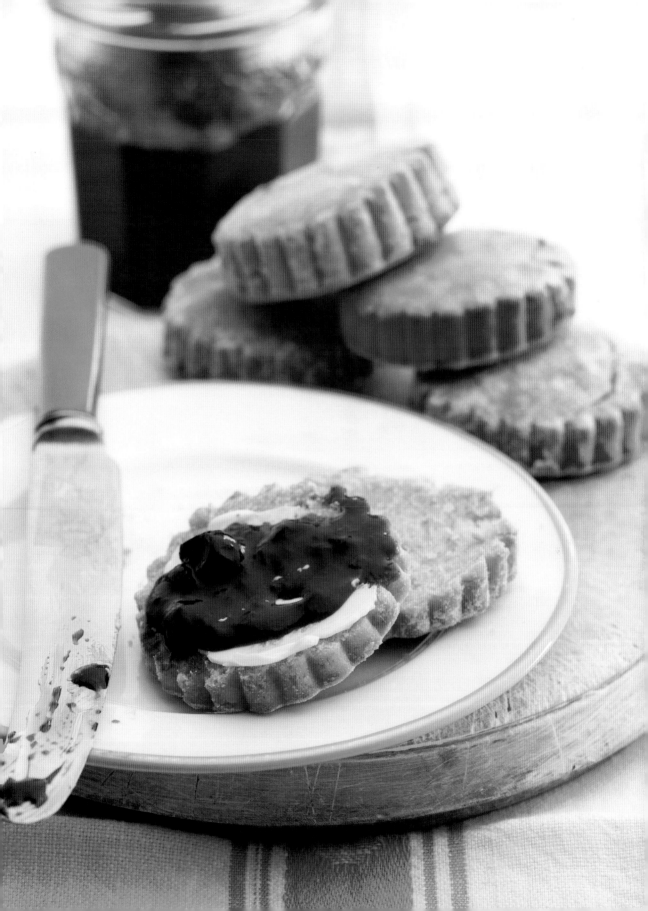

Dinners

By the time we have put my daughter, Zoë, to bed in the evening,
it's generally getting late. So I want recipes I can put together with
minimal effort—whether it's for a meal by myself or with lots of people.
Here you'll find Herb- and Olive-Crusted Lamb, for example, that you
can whip up in no time at all; or recipes you can prepare ahead and keep
in the refrigerator or freezer until needed, like the Vegetable Tagine,
the paste for the Shrimp & Butternut Squash Curry, or the batches
of sauce for the Lasagne. And you'll also find some show-stoppers that
look far more difficult to make than they actually are, such as the
Roasted Onion, Fig and Lemon Thyme Tart or Duck with Plums.

Salmon en Croûte, page 138 >

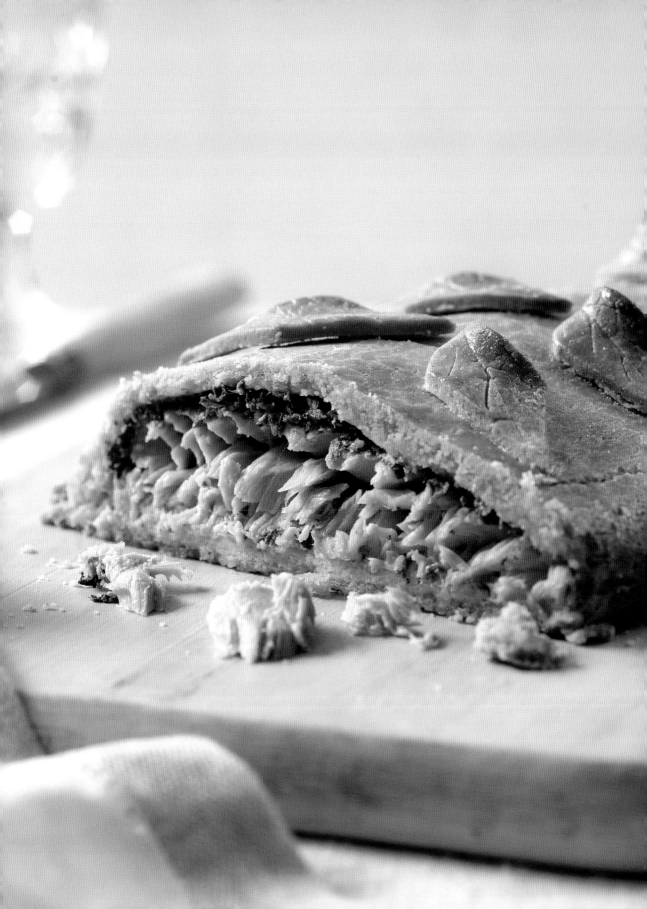

This is wonderful for a weekend dinner, or even a Sunday lunch — and you can also use the stuffing with turkey for a gluten- and dairy-free Thanksgiving meal.

Apricot- and Thyme-Stuffed Chicken

Serves **4**   Preparation time **30 minutes, plus making the stock**   Cooking time **2 hours 5 minutes**

1 cup unsulfured dried apricots, chopped

½ onion, chopped

1 garlic clove, crushed

scant 1½ cups rice flakes

3 tablespoons dairy-free margarine, diced, plus
    extra for greasing

1 teaspoon chopped thyme leaves, plus thyme
    sprigs to serve

4-pound oven-ready chicken

1 tablespoon olive oil

1 cup plus 2 tablespoons Chicken Stock
    (see page 20) or stock made from
    gluten- and dairy-free bouillon powder

1 cup plus 2 tablespoons dry white wine

1 tablespoon cornstarch

sea salt and freshly ground black pepper

1 Put the dried apricots and 1¼ cups water in a saucepan and bring to a boil over high heat. Turn the heat down to medium and simmer 15 to 20 minutes until the fruit is soft and the water is absorbed. Transfer to a large bowl and mix in the onion, garlic, rice flakes, dairy-free margarine and thyme. Season with salt and pepper.

2 Preheat the oven to 350°F. Stuff the chicken and secure the opening by threading a toothpick or small skewer through the skin, then put it in a large baking dish or deep roasting pan. Rub the oil over the chicken, season lightly with salt and pepper, and add the stock and wine. Cover with baking parchment, making sure the ends of the paper are tucked under the dish. Bake 1 hour, then remove from the oven and set aside the baking parchment.

3 Grease a small baking dish with dairy-free margarine, put any remaining stuffing in it, and cover with baking parchment, tucking the ends of the paper under the dish. Put the chicken and stuffing in the oven and bake 40 minutes longer, or until the juices run clear when the thickest part of the thigh is pierced with a skewer. If the juices look at all pink, bake a little longer. Remove both dishes from the oven and cover the chicken again with the baking parchment, tucking the ends of the paper under the dish. Let stand at room temperature 10 to 15 minutes.

4 Meanwhile, pour the pan juices into a small saucepan and bring to a boil over high heat. Put the cornstarch and 1 tablespoon water in a small bowl and stir until smooth, then stir it into the pan juices. Simmer, stirring, 2 to 3 minutes until thickened. Season with salt and pepper. Serve the chicken and stuffing with the gravy and thyme sprigs.

dinners

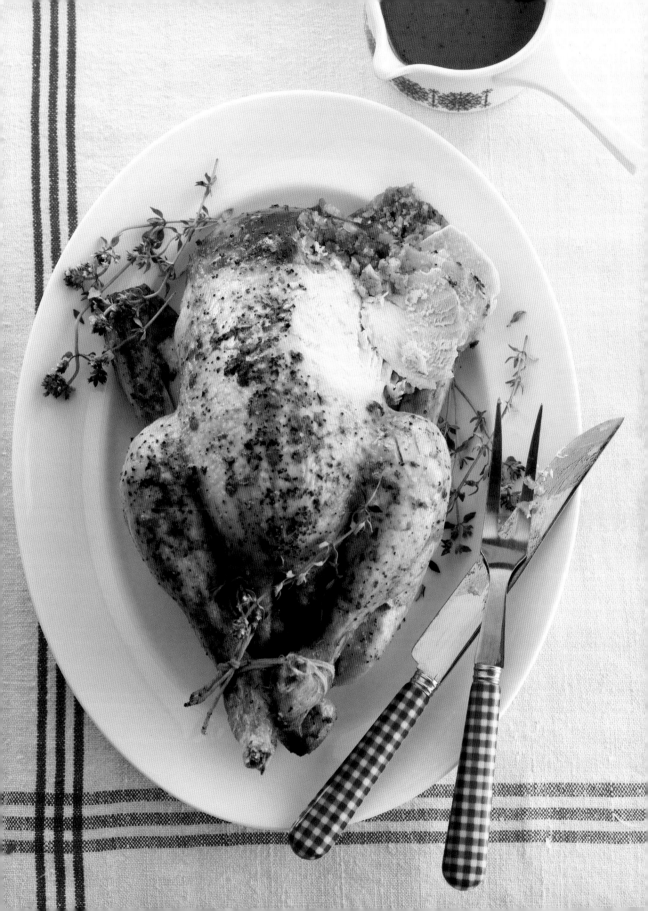

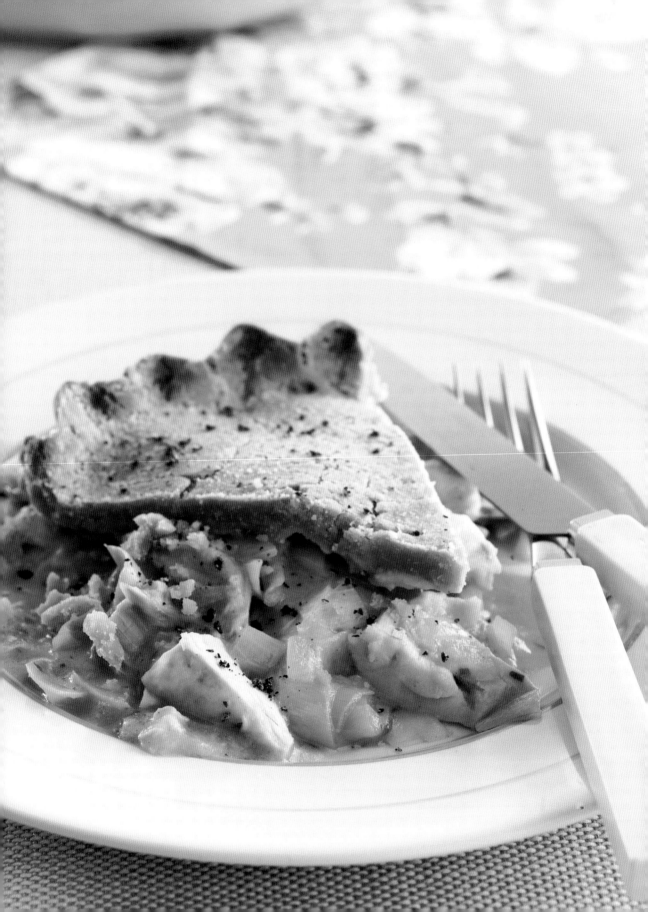

Hearty, warming, and wholesome — there's nothing like a great pot pie. Here I've used tarragon to add a subtle hint of aniseed to the chicken and leeks.

Chicken and Tarragon Pie

Serves **4** Preparation time **15 minutes, plus making the chicken, sauce, and dough**
Cooking time **55 minutes**

2 tablespoons olive oil

1 onion, chopped

1 leek, chopped

4-pound unstuffed roast chicken (see page 106),
    cut into bite-size pieces and juices reserved

1 handful of tarragon leaves, chopped

1 recipe quantity White Sauce (see page 12),
    substituting the juices from the chicken for
    some of the stock

brown rice flour, for dusting

1 recipe quantity Basic Piecrust Dough
    (see page 19)

sea salt and freshly ground black pepper

1 Preheat the oven to 400°F. Heat the oil in a large, heavy-bottomed saucepan over medium heat. Add the onion and cook, stirring occasionally, 2 to 3 minutes until just starting to turn golden, then add the leek and cook 3 to 4 minutes longer until soft.

2 Transfer to a 2-quart baking dish and stir in the chicken and tarragon. Heat the white sauce and stir it into the mixture, then season lightly with salt and pepper.

3 Liberally dust a cutting board with rice flour and roll out the dough into a circle about ⅛ inch thick, and 1¼ inches wider than the dish. Be careful because the dough will still be slightly sticky. Ease the dough onto the top of the baking dish and cover the filling. If the dough seems too fragile to lift, simply turn the cutting board over to drop the dough onto the filling. Press the edges of the dough down gently to crimp and neaten the edge, using a sharp knife. Cut a small cross in the middle to let the steam out.

4 Bake 40 to 45 minutes until the pastry is a rich, golden brown, then serve sprinkled with black pepper, if desired.

dinners

I love cashew nut cream! Here it gives thickness and creaminess to the curry and reduces the full-on heat of the spices and chilies.

Chicken Tikka Masala

Serves **4**   Preparation time **15 minutes, plus making the nut cream**   Cooking time **30 minutes**

2 tablespoons olive oil

4 boneless, skinless chicken breast halves,
    cut into bite-size pieces

½ cup tomato puree

½ recipe quantity Cashew Nut Cream
    (see page 13)

1 handful of cilantro leaves, chopped

cashew nuts, chopped, to serve

½ red chili, seeded and finely chopped,
    to serve

MASALA PASTE:

2 red chilies, seeded

3 garlic cloves

1-inch piece ginger root, peeled

1 onion, quartered

juice of ½ lemon

1 teaspoon ground cumin

1 teaspoon ground coriander

1 teaspoon turmeric

2 teaspoon garam masala

½ teaspoon cayenne pepper

1 teaspoon honey

3 tablespoons dairy-free margarine

1 small handful of cilantro leaves and stems,
    coarsely chopped

1 tablespoon tomato paste

2 tablespoons olive oil

1 Put all of the ingredients for the masala paste in a blender or food processor and blend until a smooth paste forms, then set aside.

2 Heat the oil in a large, heavy-bottomed saucepan over medium heat. Add the chicken and cook, stirring occasionally, 5 to 6 minutes until light brown. Stir in the masala paste and tomato puree, then turn the heat up to medium-high. When the mixture starts to bubble, reduce the heat to medium-low and simmer, covered, stirring occasionally, 15 to 20 minutes until the chicken is cooked through.

3 Stir in the nut cream and simmer, stirring frequently, 3 to 4 minutes longer until heated through. Add a little water if the mixture becomes too dry. Sprinkle with the cilantro leaves, cashew nuts, and extra chilli and serve.

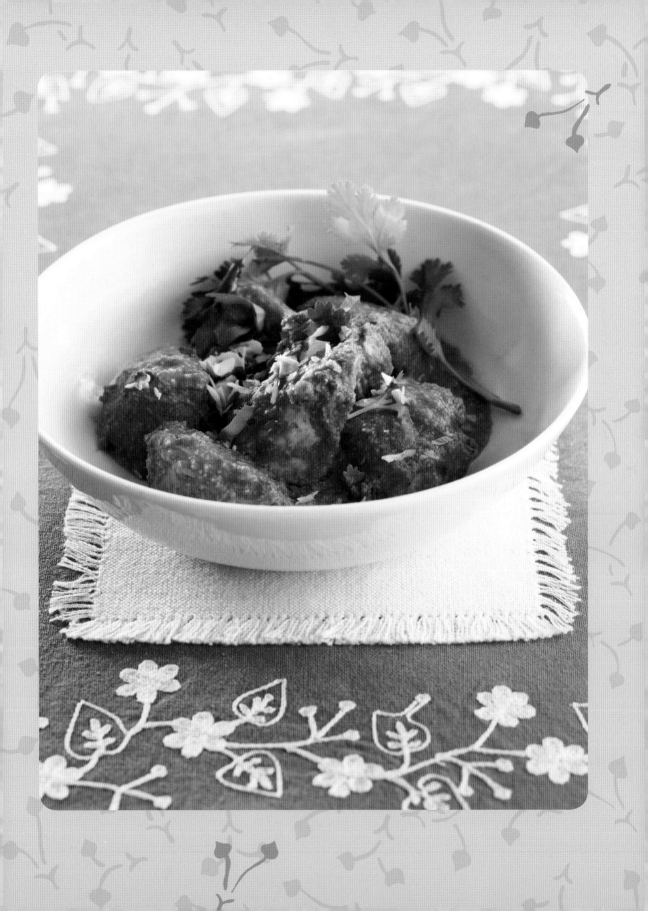

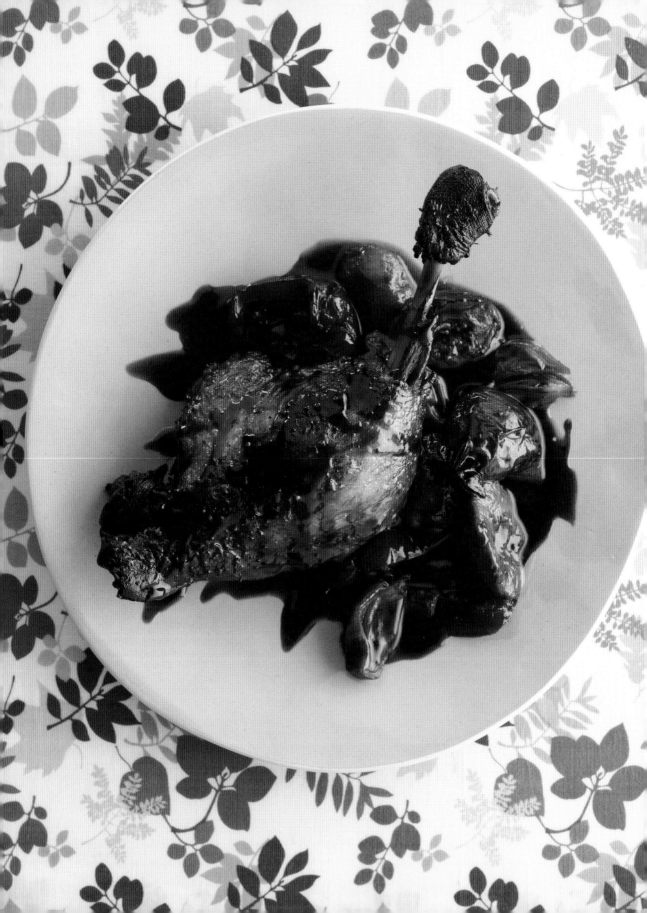

*Umeboshi paste is made from pickled ume fruit, a type of Japanese plum.
They have been called the kings of alkaline foods and help your body to digest
foods properly and absorb nutrients fully.*

Duck with Plums

Serves **4**   Preparation time **10 minutes, plus at least 2 hours marinating**
Cooking time **2 hours 50 minutes**

4 duck legs

8 shallots

16 plums, halved and pitted

**3 red, orange, or yellow bell peppers, seeded
    and quartered**

sea salt and freshly ground black pepper

MARINADE:

2 tablespoons olive oil

¼ cup tamari soy sauce

1 tablespoon umeboshi paste

¼ cup honey

3 star anise

1 cinnamon stick

1   Put the duck legs, meat-side down, in an ovenproof casserole or baking dish just large
enough to fit them. Whisk together all of the ingredients for the marinade and pour it
over the duck. Cover with a lid and let marinate in the refrigerator at least 2 hours,
preferably overnight.

2   Preheat the oven to 315°F. Remove the duck from the refrigerator and, lifting the legs up
as needed, put the shallots, plums, and peppers on the bottom of the dish. Turn the duck
legs meat-side up and season lightly with salt and pepper. Bake, covered, 2 hours and
15 minutes, or until the meat is tender.

3   Remove the casserole from the oven and transfer the duck legs to a plate. Pour most of the
juices from the casserole into a saucepan, discarding the cinnamon and star anise, and bring
to a boil over high heat. Turn the heat down to medium-high and simmer 15 to 20 minutes
until it is reduced by about half. Meanwhile, put the duck back in the casserole and bake,
uncovered, 15 minutes longer. Remove from the oven and serve with the sauce.

dinners

This gluten-free version of the traditional slow-cooked recipe uses chorizo and pancetta instead of sausages, giving it an extra depth and richness.

Pork and Duck Cassoulet

Serves **4** Preparation time **10 minutes, plus 12 hours soaking (optional) and making the stock**
Cooking time **4 hours 45 minutes**

1 cup dried haricot or navy beans or 1½ cups
    drained canned haricot beans, rinsed
2 duck legs
1 tablespoon olive oil
5 ounces pancetta
1 pound pork tenderloin, cut into large cubes
2 tablespoons goose fat
1 onion, finely sliced
4 garlic cloves, crushed

1 carrot, diced
2 bay leaves
heaped 1 tablespoon thyme leaves
heaped 1 tablespoon chopped rosemary leaves
2 handfuls of flat-leaf parsley leaves, chopped
2⅔ cups Vegetable Stock (see page 21) or
    vegetable stock made from gluten- and
    dairy-free bouillon powder
8 ounces chorizo, skinned and sliced

1   If using dried beans, put them in a bowl, cover with cold water, and soak overnight, or at least 12 hours, then drain and rinse well. Transfer to a large saucepan, cover with fresh water, and bring to a boil over high heat. Boil rapidly 10 minutes, then turn the heat down to medium-low, cover with a lid, and simmer 1 hour, or until tender. Drain well.

2   Preheat the oven to 400°F. Put the duck legs in a small roasting pan and roast 30 minutes. Remove from the oven and turn the oven down to 275°F.

3   Heat the oil in a large, heavy-bottomed saucepan over medium heat. Add the pancetta and fry, stirring occasionally, 3 to 4 minutes until crisp, then remove, using a slotted spoon, and set aside. Add the pork to the pan and cook, turning occasionally, 5 minutes until brown. Remove, using a slotted spoon, and set aside with the pancetta.

4   Melt the goose fat in the pan, then add the onion. Cook, stirring occasionally, 2 to 3 minutes until just starting to turn golden. Stir in the garlic and cook about 30 seconds, then add the carrot and herbs and cook 2 minutes longer. Add the stock and bring to a boil over high heat, then lower the heat to medium and simmer 2 minutes.

5   Skin the duck, then put it in an ovenproof casserole. Add the pancetta, pork, chorizo, and beans. Add the stock mixture, stir well, and cook, uncovered, 3 hours. Remove the bones after 2 hours, stir and cook 1 hour longer. Remove the bay leaves and serve.

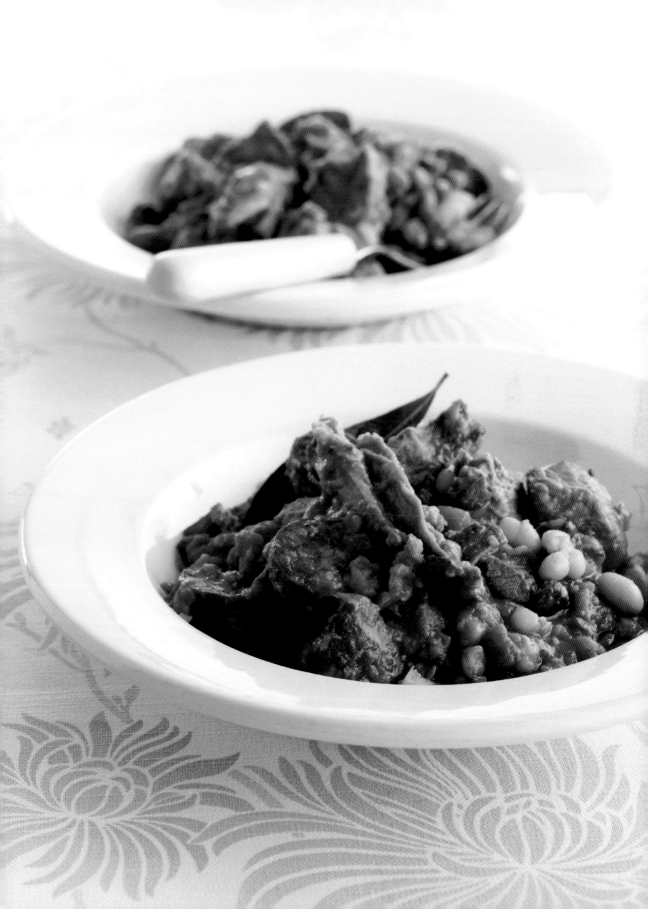

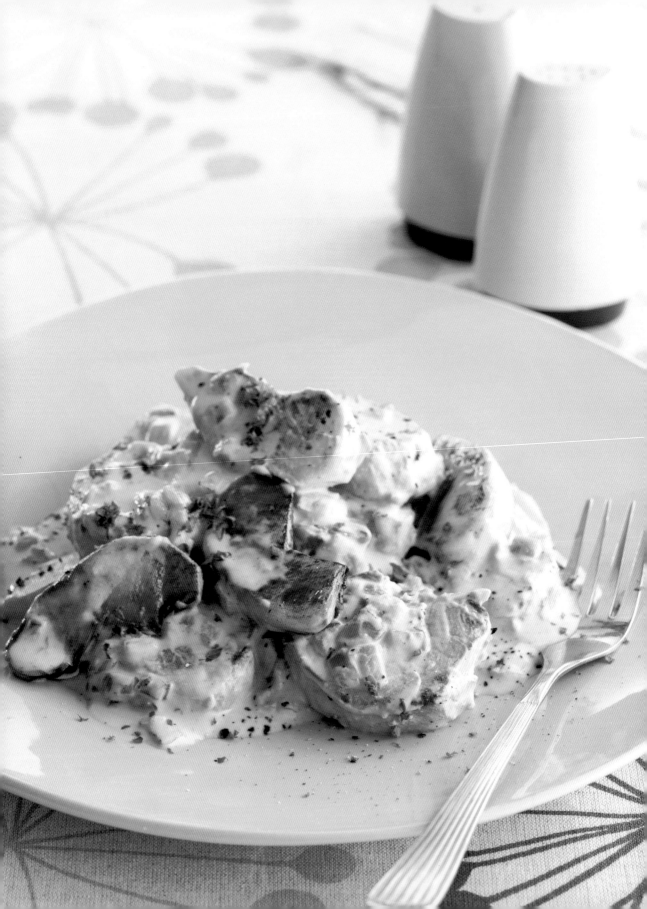

Soy cream has a fairly distinctive taste, but here the flavors of the pork, apple, lemon, and white wine combine with it to create a delicious dish.

Pork in a Creamy Apple Sauce

Serves **4**   Preparation time **15 minutes**   Cooking time **20 minutes**

3½ tablespoons dairy-free margarine

1 pound 10 ounces pork tenderloin, trimmed
    of fat and cut into bite-size chunks

3 apples

juice of ½ lemon

1 onion, finely chopped

1 garlic clove, crushed

scant ½ cup dry white wine

½ cup soy cream

sea salt and freshly ground black pepper

1   Heat the dairy-free margarine in a large, heavy-bottomed saucepan over medium heat. Add the pork and cook, stirring frequently, 5 to 6 minutes until well brown on all sides. Remove from the pan, using a slotted spoon, and set aside.

2   Peel the apples, then cut them into quarters and remove the cores. Slice each quarter into 3 slices and dip into the lemon juice.

3   Put the onion in the saucepan and fry over low heat, stirring occasionally, 2 minutes until just turning golden. Stir in the garlic, then add the apple slices and cook 2 to 3 minutes, stirring occasionally, until golden. Return the pork to the pan and add the wine. Bring to a boil over high heat, then reduce the heat to medium and simmer 5 minutes. Stir in the soy cream, season lightly with salt and pepper, and cook 2 to 3 minutes longer. Serve hot.

dinners

Amaranth is a fantastic gluten-free alternative to couscous. High in iron, calcium, and protein, it also contains important phytonutrients that boost your immune system.

Lamb Burgers with Pomegranate Amaranth

Serves **4**   Preparation time **20 minutes**   Cooking time **40 minutes**

1¼ cups amaranth

2 pomegranates

1 pound 12 ounces ground lamb

1 red onion, finely chopped

2 garlic cloves, crushed

½ teaspoon crushed chili flakes

1 tablespoon pomegranate molasses

2 large handfuls of flat-leaf parsley leaves, chopped

5 tablespoons olive oil

⅔ cup pistachios, coarsely chopped

1 handful of mint leaves, chopped

juice of 2 lemons

sea salt

1   Put the amaranth and 3¼ cups cold water in a saucepan and bring to a boil over high heat. Turn the heat down to medium and simmer, covered, 15 to 20 minutes until the amaranth is tender and the water is absorbed. Add a little more water during cooking, if needed. Set aside.

2   Halve the pomegranates and set 3 of the halves aside. Hold the remaining half over a large bowl, bash the outer skin with a wooden spoon until all of the seeds fall out into the bowl. You'll need to bash the skin a few times before the seeds start to fall out, but they will. Put the ground lamb, onion, garlic, chili flakes, pomegranate molasses, and a small handful of the parsley in the bowl. Season with salt and mix well. Using your hands, divide the mixture into 8 equal pieces and shape each one into a burger.

3   Heat 1 tablespoon of the oil in a large, heavy-bottomed skillet over medium heat. Add half of the burgers and cook about 5 minutes on each side, or until they are cooked to your liking. Remove from the pan, set aside and repeat with the remaining burgers and another 1 tablespoon of the oil.

4   Bash the outer skins of the remaining halves of the pomegranates over another large bowl. Add the pistachios, mint leaves, lemon juice, amaranth, and remaining oil to the bowl and mix well. Serve with the burgers.

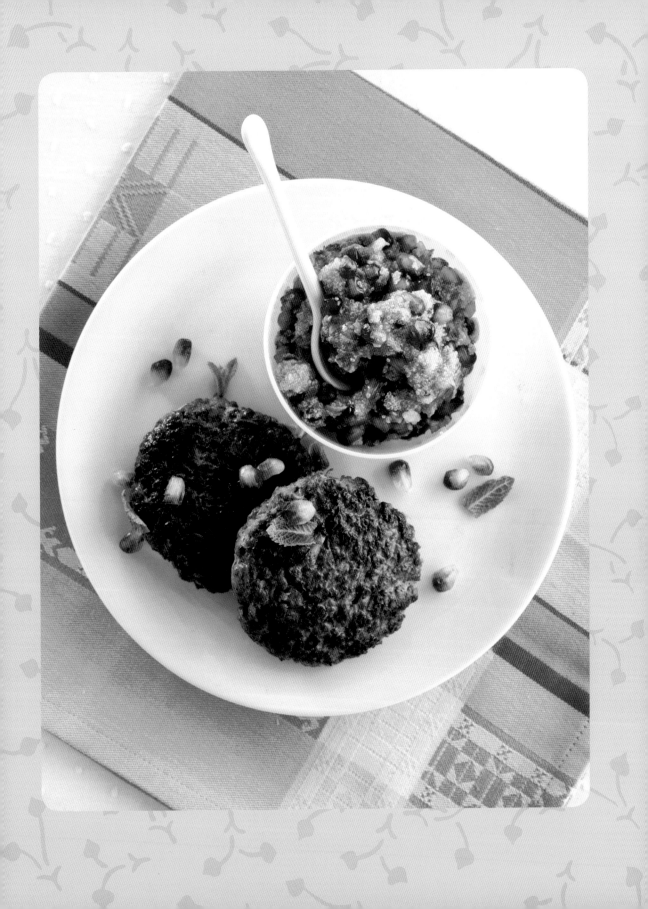

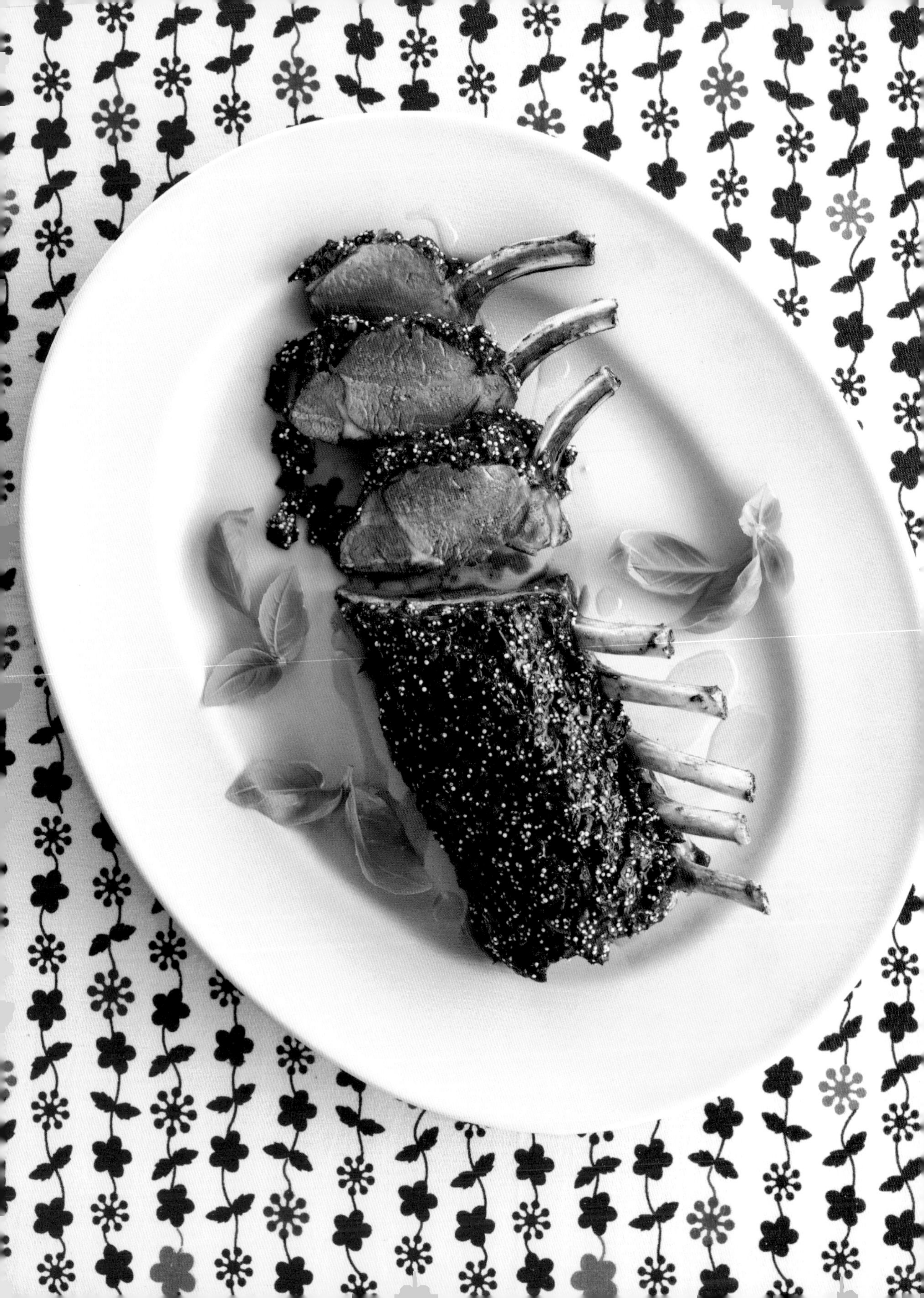

I've used anchovies for flavor in this recipe but they're also a great source of vitamins and minerals — and, more importantly, of omega-3.

Herb- and Olive- Crusted Lamb

Serves **4**   Preparation time **25 minutes**   Cooking time **30 minutes**

¼ cup capers in salt or brine

2 French-trimmed racks of lamb, each with
    8 cutlets

3 tablespoons olive oil

1 ounce drained anchovies in oil

½ cup drained black olives in brine

2 garlic cloves

1 tablespoon tomato paste

1 handful of parsley leaves, coarsely chopped

1 small handful of basil leaves

1   Preheat the oven to 400°F. Rinse the capers and soak them in a bowl of water 10 minutes, then rinse and drain well. If using capers in brine, just rinse and drain them.

2   Meanwhile, score the layer of fat on each rack of lamb. Heat 1 tablespoon of the oil in a heavy-bottomed skillet over a medium-high heat. Add the lamb and sear 2 minutes on each side until brown all over, then transfer to a roasting pan, fat-side up.

3   Put the capers, anchovies, olives, garlic, tomato paste, parsley, basil, and amaranth in a food processor and blend to form a finely chopped paste. With the motor running, add the remaining oil and blend until well combined. Spoon the mixture over the top of the fat, pressing down well with the back of the spoon.

4   Bake 20 to 25 minutes, depending on how pink you like the meat. Remove the racks of lamb from the oven and cover with baking parchment, ensuring the ends of the paper are tucked under the pan. Let stand 5 minutes, then remove the baking parchment and serve.

dinners

Instead of a cooked herb crust, the steaks in this recipe are coated with fresh herbs. Their punchy flavors brighten up the dish and meld beautifully with the mushroom sauce.

Herb-Rolled Steak with Mushroom Sauce

Serves **4**   Preparation time **35 minutes**   Cooking time **20 minutes**

1 handful of mint leaves, finely chopped

1 handful of cilantro leaves, finely chopped

1 large handful of flat-leaf parsley leaves, finely chopped

1 tablespoon olive oil

4 beef filet steaks

sea salt and freshly ground black pepper

MUSHROOM SAUCE:

1 ounce mixed dried mushrooms, such as shiitake and porcini

1 tablespoon dairy-free margarine

2 shallots, finely chopped

1 tablespoon brandy

scant 1 cup dry white wine

¼ cup soy cream

dinners

1   To make the sauce, put the mushrooms and 1¼ cups cold water in a bowl and soak for 20 minutes. Strain through a sieve into a clean bowl and reserve the liquid.

2   Heat the dairy-free margarine in a heavy-bottomed saucepan over low heat. Add the shallots and fry, stirring occasionally, 1 to 2 minutes until just starting to turn golden. Stir in the soaked mushrooms and cook 2 minutes longer, then add the brandy, followed by the wine and the reserved mushroom liquid. Bring to a boil over high heat, then reduce the heat to medium and simmer 15 minutes, or until reduced by about half.

3   Meanwhile, mix the mint, cilantro, and parsley leaves together in a bowl and set aside. Heat the oil in a large, heavy-bottomed skillet over medium heat. Season the steaks lightly with salt and pepper, add them to the pan and cook 3 to 4 minutes on each side for medium-rare or 1 to 2 minutes longer for well done. Alternatively, brush the steaks with the remaining oil and cook under a hot broiler.

4   Blend the sauce to a puree in a blender. Stir in the soy cream, season lightly with salt and pepper, and cook 1 minute longer.

5   Roll the steaks in the herbs, covering them as much as possible. Serve immediately with the mushroom sauce.

Slow-cooking gives you the opportunity to use cheaper cuts of meat, yet still end up with wonderfully tender results.

Slow-Cooked Beef

Serves **4**   Preparation time **15 minutes, plus making the stock**   Cooking time **3 hours 40 minutes**

2 tablespoons olive oil

1 pound 12 ounces casserole beef, cut into
   chunks

2 onions, finely chopped

2 large garlic cloves, crushed

3¼ cups dry red wine

1 cup plus 2 tablespoons Vegetable Stock
   (see page 21) or vegetable stock made from
   gluten- and dairy-free bouillon powder

1 ounce dried porcini mushrooms

2 bay leaves

1 tablespoon finely chopped rosemary leaves

1 tablespoon finely chopped thyme leaves

2 tablespoons kuzu

sea salt and freshly ground black pepper

1   Heat the oil in a large, heavy-bottomed skillet over medium heat. Add the steak and cook,
    stirring occasionally, 5 minutes, or until lightly browned. Remove the beef from the pan with
    a slotted spoon, transfer to an ovenproof casserole, and set aside.

2   Preheat the oven to 300°F. Add the onions to the pan and cook, stirring occasionally, for
    2 to 3 minutes until starting to turn golden, then stir in the garlic. Add the red wine, stock,
    porcini mushrooms, bay leaves, rosemary, and thyme and season lightly with salt. Cover and
    bring to a boil over high heat. Pour the mixture into the casserole and stir. Transfer to the
    oven and cook, covered, 3½ hours, or until the beef is tender.

3   Ladle most of the liquid from the casserole into a saucepan and heat over medium heat.
    In a small bowl, mix the kuzu and 2 tablespoons cold water together to make a paste. Stir
    the mixture into the pan and simmer, stirring occasionally, 2 to 3 minutes longer until
    thickened. Season lightly with salt and pepper and remove the bay leaves. Stir the sauce into
    the beef and serve.

dinners

A gluten-free, dairy-free version of one of the all-time family favorites — my little angel, Zoë, adores this!

Lasagne

Serves **4**   Preparation time **10 minutes, plus making the sauces**   Cooking time **1 hour**

1 recipe quantity Roasted Tomato and Pepper
  Sauce (see page 12)
1 small handful of flat-leaf parsley leaves,
  chopped, plus extra to serve
1 pound 2 ounces ground steak

1½ recipe quantities White Sauce (see page 12)
2 cups shredded soy cheese
¼ teaspoon freshly grated nutmeg
12 no-precook gluten-free lasagne sheets

1   Preheat the oven to 350°F. Heat the roasted tomato and pepper sauce in a large
    heavy-bottomed saucepan over medium-low heat and add the parsley. Crumble in the
    ground steak and simmer 8 to 10 minutes.

2   Put the white sauce in another saucepan, stir in the soy cheese and the nutmeg, and heat
    over low heat.

3   Spread one-third of the tomato sauce over the bottom of a 9- x 7-inch baking dish, then
    drizzle one-quarter of the cheese sauce over the top and cover with a layer of 6 lasagne
    sheets. Layer again with the tomato sauce, cheese sauce, and 6 lasagne sheets. Cover with
    the remaining tomato sauce and the remaining cheese sauce, making sure the cheese sauce
    covers everything on top.

4   Bake 45 to 50 minutes, depending on the type of lasagne sheets used, until the cheese sauce
    is golden brown and the pasta is soft. Sprinkle with parsley and serve hot.

dinners

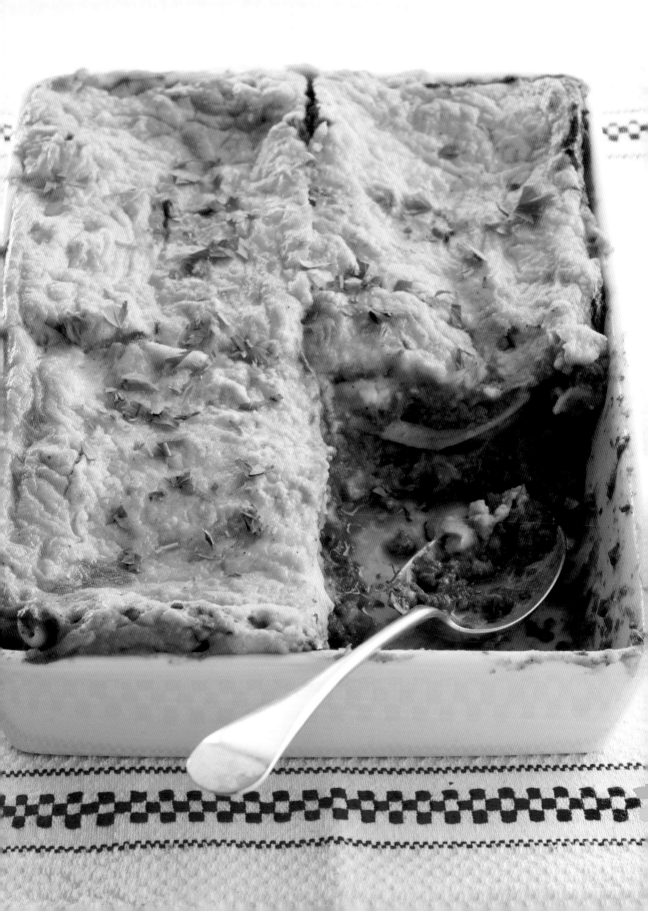

Fiery and fresh, this curry combines sweetness from the butternut squash and coconut and sourness from the kaffir lime leaves, lemongrass, and lime.

Shrimp and Butternut Squash Curry

Serves **4**   Preparation time **15 minutes**   Cooking time **30 minutes**

1 tablespoon olive oil

1 cup plus 2 tablespoons coconut cream

1¾ cups coconut milk

1 tablespoon tamari soy sauce

1 to 2 tablespoons Thai fish sauce

1 pound 2 ounces butternut squash, peeled and
    cut into ¾-inch cubes

1 pound 2 ounces cooked jumbo shrimp

juice of 1 lime

1 small handful of cilantro leaves,
    to serve

CURRY PASTE:

½ teaspoon cumin seeds

½ teaspoon coriander seeds

1 red chili, coarsely chopped

2 shallots, coarsely chopped

2 garlic cloves, coarsely chopped

1-inch piece of ginger root, peeled and
    coarsely chopped

2 kaffir lime leaves

1 lemongrass stalk, coarsely chopped

½ teaspoon shrimp paste

zest of 1 lime

1 handful of cilantro leaves and stems, coarsely
    chopped, plus extra sprigs to serve

1 To make the curry paste, heat a heavy-bottomed skillet over low heat. Add the cumin and coriander seeds and cook, stirring continuously, 2 to 3 minutes until fragrant. Remove the seeds from the heat and grind to a fine powder with a mini food processor or spice mill. Add the chili, shallots, garlic, and ginger and blend well, then add all of the remaining ingredients for the paste and blend to form a coarse paste. Set aside.

2 Heat a wok or large skillet over medium heat until hot. Add the oil and swirl it around, then turn the heat down to low and add the coconut cream and coconut milk. Cook over low heat 4 to 5 minutes. Add the curry paste and cook 2 to 3 minutes, stirring well.

3 Add the tamari, 1 tablespoon of the fish sauce, and the squash and cook over medium heat 12 to 15 minutes until the squash is tender. Take care not to let the mixture boil or the coconut milk will curdle. Stir in the shrimp and cook 2 to 3 minutes until they are hot, then stir in the lime juice. Check the seasoning and add a little more fish sauce to taste if needed. Sprinkle with the chopped cilantro and serve with extra cilantro sprigs.

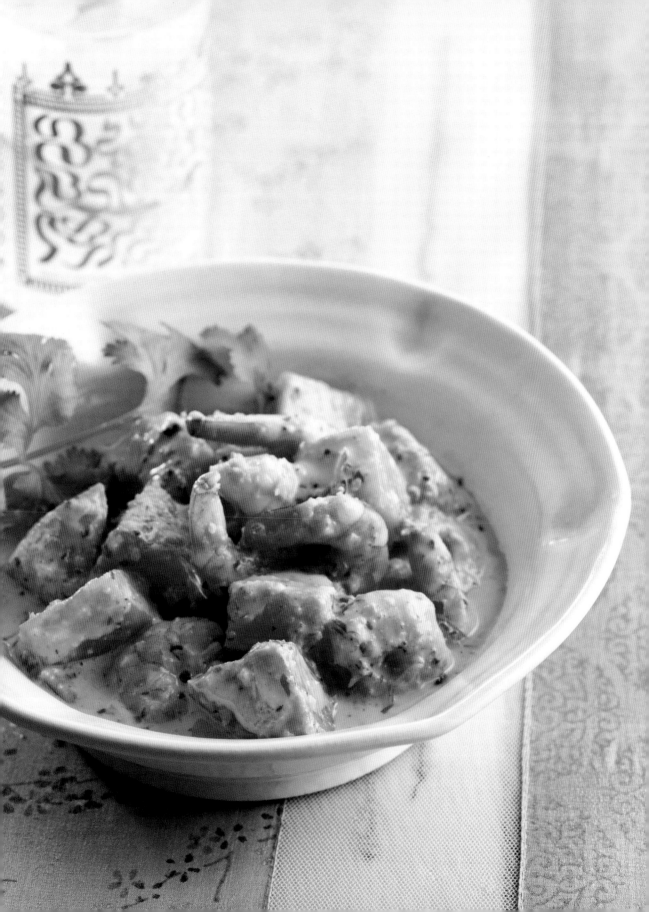

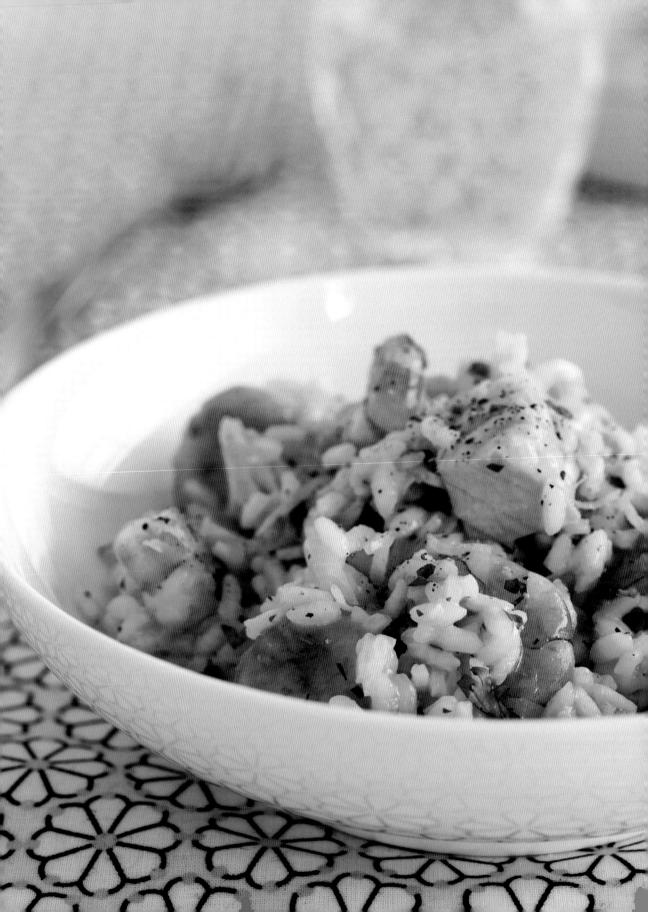

Not your standard risotto—this one combines the rich, sweet flavors of seafood with lemon zest and parsley to give it a herby, zingy freshness.

Seafood Risotto

Serves **4**   Preparation time **15 minutes, plus making the stock**   Cooking time **35 minutes**

3½ cups Vegetable Stock (see page 21) or
    vegetable stock made from gluten- and
    dairy-free bouillon powder

a pinch of saffron strands

¼ cup olive oil

1 onion, finely chopped

2 garlic cloves, crushed

1¼ cups dry white wine

10 ounces boneless, skinless salmon, cut into
    bite-size pieces

1¼ cups arborio or other risotto rice

9 ounces small scallops (or larger ones, cut in
    half horizontally), removed from their shells

9 ounces raw jumbo shrimp

zest of 1 lemon

1 handful of parsley leaves, chopped

sea salt and freshly ground black pepper

1 Put the stock in a saucepan and bring to a boil over medium heat. Remove from the heat, add the saffron, and set aside.

2 Heat 2 tablespoons of the oil in a large, heavy-bottomed saucepan over medium heat. Add the onion and cook, stirring occasionally, 2 to 3 minutes until just starting to turn golden. Stir in the garlic and cook about 30 seconds, then stir in the wine and bring to a boil over high heat. Lower the heat to medium, add the salmon and poach 5 minutes, or until cooked through. Remove the salmon with a slotted spoon and set aside.

3 Add the rice to the onion mixture and add 1 ladleful of the hot stock. Cook over medium-low heat, stirring continuously, until all of the liquid is absorbed. Continue stirring in ladlefuls of the hot stock until almost all of the liquid is absorbed. This will take 18 to 20 minutes.

4 Meanwhile, put the remaining oil in a skillet over medium heat, add the scallops, and fry 1 to 2 minutes on each side until golden brown or no longer translucent. Remove from the pan and transfer to a plate. Add the shrimp to the pan and fry, turning occasionally, 2 to 3 minutes until pink and cooked through. Remove from the pan and set aside with the scallops.

5 When the risotto is almost cooked, add the fish and seafood and season lightly with salt and pepper. Stir in the lemon zest and cook 2 minutes longer until the rice is soft but still has a slight bite, the fish and seafood are hot, and all the liquid is absorbed. Stir in the parsley and serve immediately.

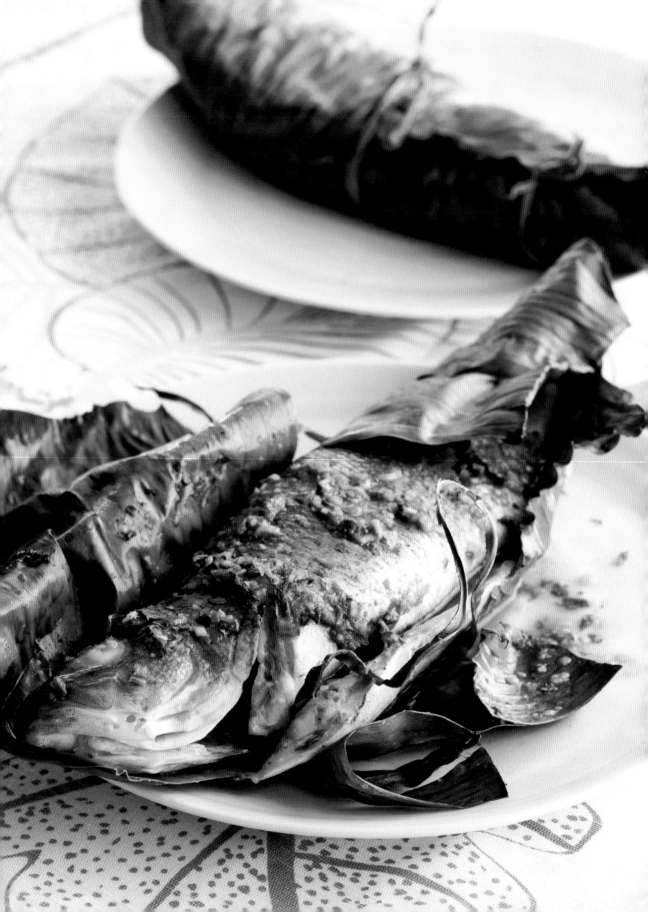

Cooking with banana leaves is a fantastic alternative to using aluminum foil, which contains heavy metals. They're available in many Asian grocery stores, but if you can't find any, you can use baking parchment instead.

Roasted Sea Bass in Banana Leaf

Serves **4**   Preparation time **15 minutes, plus 2 hours marinating**   Cooking time **15 minutes**

2 tablespoons olive oil

2 tablespoons tamari soy sauce

juice of 1 lime

1 tablespoon agave syrup

1 teaspoon shrimp paste

1 teaspoon freshly grated nutmeg

2 shallots, coarsely chopped

4 garlic cloves, coarsely chopped

3 lemongrass stalks, coarsely chopped

1-inch piece of ginger root, peeled and
   coarsely chopped

2 red chilies, seeded and coarsely chopped

1 handful of mint leaves, plus extra to serve

1 handful of basil leaves

2 handfuls of cilantro leaves and stems, plus
   extra leaves to serve

4 whole sea bass, dressed

2 banana leaves, cut in half

1   Put all of the ingredients, except the mint, basil, coriander, sea bass, and banana leaves, in a food processor. Blend to form a coarse, liquidy paste. Add the herbs and blend well.

2   Put a spoonful of the mixture in the cavity of each of the sea bass and put the fish in a nonmetallic dish. Spoon the remaining mixture over the fish, cover, and let marinate in the refrigerator 2 hours.

3   Preheat the oven to 350°F. Wash the banana leaves in cold water and lay one on a clean work surface. Put 1 of the sea bass on top, drizzle with a couple of spoonfuls of the marinade, and wrap securely, fastening with string, if necessary. Repeat with the remaining banana leaves and fish, then put them on a baking tray. Roast the sea bass 15 minutes, then serve.

dinners

Soy cream cheese is an excellent dairy-free ingredient that gives this dish smooth richness and great flavor.

Salmon Roulade

Serves **4 to 6**   Preparation time **20 minutes**   Cooking time **1 hour 5 minutes**

14 ounces boneless, skinless salmon

dairy-free margarine, for greasing

1 tablespoon olive oil

2 shallots, finely chopped

1 recipe quantity White Sauce (see page 12), made with 2 cups plus 2 tablespoons unsweetened soy milk instead of stock

4 eggs, separated

zest of 1 lemon

juice of ½ lemon, plus extra wedges to serve

1 ounce dill, chopped, plus extra to serve

¼ cup plus 1 teaspoon soy cream cheese

1 pound 2 ounces smoked salmon slices

sea salt and freshly ground black pepper

1   Preheat the oven to 350°F. Put the salmon in a baking dish, cover with a lid, and bake 20 to 25 minutes until cooked through, then set aside to cool. Grease a 12- x 8-inch baking tray with dairy-free margarine and line the bottom with baking parchment.

2   Heat the oil in a large, heavy-bottomed saucepan over low heat. Add the shallots and cook, stirring occasionally, 2 to 3 minutes until they start to turn golden. In another heavy-bottomed saucepan, heat the white sauce over medium heat, then remove from the heat and whisk in the egg yolks. Fold in the shallots and season lightly with salt and pepper.

3   Put the egg whites in a clean bowl and whisk until stiff peaks form. Add one-third of them to the egg-yolk mixture and whisk until blended. With a metal spoon, fold in the remaining egg whites until well mixed. Pour the mixture into the baking tray and bake 25 minutes, or until golden brown.

4   Meanwhile, put the cooked salmon, lemon zest and juice, dill, and soy cream cheese in a food processor, season lightly with salt and pepper, bearing in mind that the smoked salmon will be salty, and blend well.

5   Remove the baked egg mixture from the oven and let cool a few minutes. Remove it from the baking tray and remove the baking parchment. Turn it over and put it on a clean dish towel. Cover with a layer of smoked salmon, then spoon the cooked salmon mixture over the top and spread evenly. Using the dish towel to hold the bottom, carefully roll the long side of the roulade over until it forms a large, thick rope shape. Serve warm with lemon wedges and sprinkled with dill and black pepper, or leave it to cool, then wrap it in plastic wrap and chill in the refrigerator up to 12 hours before serving.

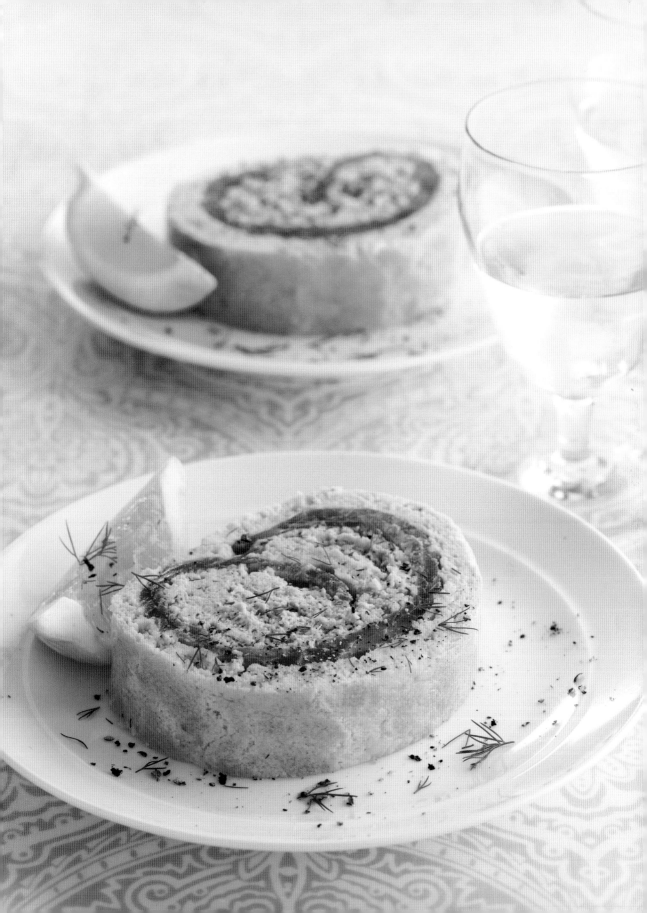

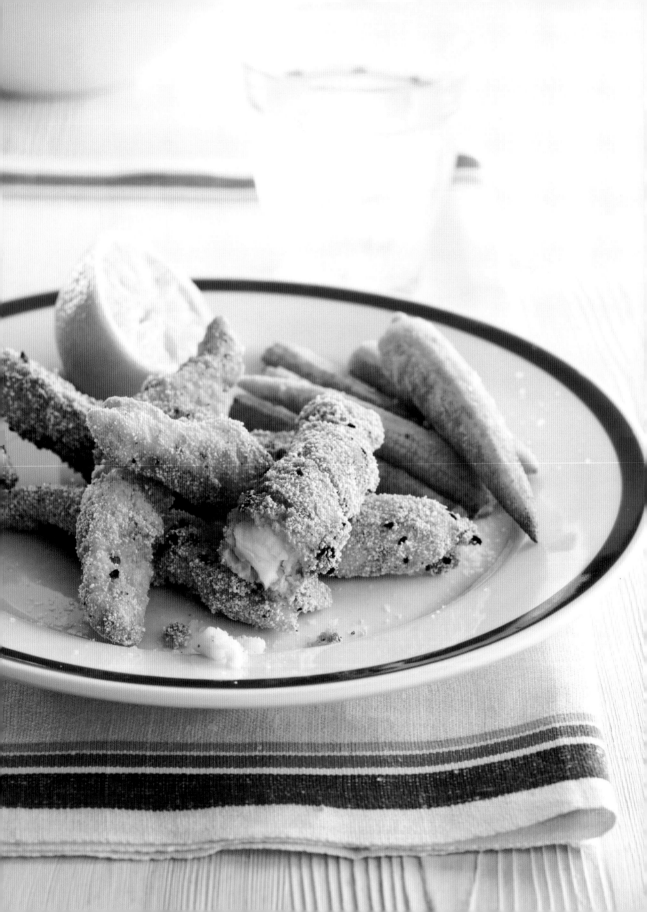

The combination of cornstarch and polenta makes a lovely crisp, crunchy coating for the fish — and the rice flour gives the corn a delicate crunch.

Fish Goujons with Crispy Baby Corn

Serves **4**   Preparation time **15 minutes**   Cooking time **10 minutes**

⅔ cup cornstarch

2 extra-large eggs

1⅓ cups fast-cook polenta

1 teaspoon crushed chili flakes

4 ounces boneless, skinless white fish fillets,
    such as cod, sliced into strips

2 cups canola oil

sea salt and freshly ground black pepper

CRISPY BABY CORN:

10 ounces baby corn cobs

¼ cup soy milk

⅔ cup rice flour

1 cup canola oil

1   For the crispy baby corn, put the corn in a steamer and steam, covered, over high heat 5 to 6 minutes until just tender but still crunchy, then set aside. Put the soy milk and rice flour in two separate bowls and season the rice flour with salt and pepper, then set aside.

2   Put the cornstarch, eggs, and polenta in three separate bowls. Lightly beat the eggs. Season the polenta with the chili flakes and salt and pepper and mix well.

3   Dip each fish strip into the cornstarch to coat well, then dip it in the eggs and then in the polenta. Transfer the goujons to a plate.

4   Dip each baby corn into the soy milk and then into the rice flour to coat well. Transfer the corn cobs to another plate.

5   Heat both quantities of oil in separate large saucepans or woks until very hot. To test if the oil is hot enough, drop 1 baby corn into the smaller quantity of oil. It should sizzle and begin to brown immediately. If not, remove it and let the oil heat some more. When the oil is hot enough, quickly put half of the fish goujons in the larger quantity of hot oil and half of the corn in the other, working in batches to avoid overcrowding the pans. Deep-fry the fish 2 minutes, or until golden brown and cooked through. Deep-fry the corn 1½ to 2 minutes, turning half way through, until lightly golden. Remove the fish and corn from the oils, using a slotted spoon, and drain on paper towels. Serve immediately.

dinners

If you've struggled to find a recipe that works for cheaper, more-sustainable types of fish, such as coley and pollack, this is the answer.

Fish Stew

Serves **4 to 6**   Preparation time **20 minutes, plus making the stock**   Cooking time **30 minutes**

2 tablespoons olive oil

1 onion, finely chopped

4 garlic cloves, crushed

2 fennel bulbs, chopped

2 celery sticks, chopped

2 plum tomatoes, chopped

1 pound 2 ounces mussels

½ teaspoon cayenne pepper

a pinch of saffron strands

1 tablespoon tomato paste

¾ cup dry white wine

1½ cups Fish Stock (see page 20) or
**   stock made from gluten- and dairy-free**
**   bouillon powder, heated**

2 pounds 4 ounces boneless, skinless white fish
**   fillets, cut into large chunks**

1 large handful of flat-leaf parsley leaves,
**   chopped**

sea salt and freshly ground black pepper

1   Heat the oil in a large, heavy-bottomed saucepan or deep skillet over low heat. Add the onion and cook, stirring occasionally, 2 to 3 minutes until starting to turn golden. Stir in the garlic and cook 30 seconds, then add the fennel, celery, and tomatoes. Turn the heat up to medium and cook, stirring occasionally, 10 minutes, or until the tomatoes soften a little.

2   Meanwhile, thoroughly scrub the mussels under cold running water and rinse well. Remove the beards by pulling them toward the large part of the shell. If any of the mussels are open, tap them hard against a work surface and if they don't close, discard them.

3   Stir the cayenne pepper, saffron, and tomato paste into the vegetables, then add the wine and stock. Season with salt and pepper, cover with a lid, and bring to a boil over medium-high heat. Turn the heat down to low and cook for 5 minutes until the fennel has softened.

4   Gently stir in the fish and cook 5 minutes longer, then add the mussels and press down gently so they are immersed as much as possible. Cover the pan and cook 3 minutes, then remove and discard any mussels that haven't opened. Carefully stir in the parsley and serve.

dinners

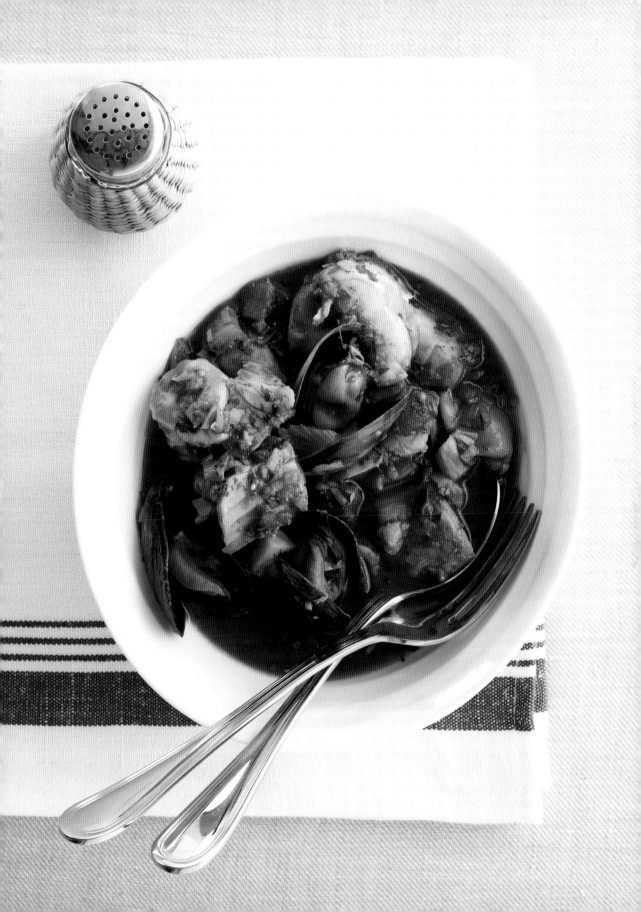

This is a wonderful recipe for entertaining — you can make the dough ahead of time and then simply whiz the herb paste together, spread it on the salmon, and create a stunning dish effortlessly.

Salmon en Croûte

Serves **4**   Preparation time **15 minutes, plus making the dough**   Cooking time **30 minutes**

3 tablespoons plus 1 teaspoon dairy-free
    margarine, plus extra for greasing

1 large handful of arugula leaves

1 small handful of mint leaves

zest of 1 lemon

½ teaspoon fine sea salt

brown rice flour, for dusting

1 recipe quantity Shortcrust Pastry Dough
    (see page 19)

1 pound 2 ounces skinned and boned
    salmon fillet

1 egg, beaten

1   Preheat the oven to 400°F. Grease a baking tray with dairy-free margarine and cut a piece of baking parchment the same size as the tray. Put the dairy-free margarine, arugula and mint leaves, lemon zest, and salt in a food processor and blend well.

2   Liberally dust a cutting board with rice flour and roll out the dough into a large rectangle about ⅛ inch thick, and slightly more than twice the width of the salmon fillet. Be careful as the dough will still be slightly sticky. Put the baking parchment over the dough and hold it in place with one hand. Turn the board over and carefully put the baking parchment, with the dough on top of it, on the work surface.

3   Put the salmon in the middle of the dough and spread the herb mixture over it. With a sharp knife, cut a 1¼- to 1½-inch square of dough away from each corner of the dough. Discard these pieces or use them to decorate the top of the dough, if desired. Using the baking parchment to keep the dough together, fold the two long sides of dough over the salmon so the edges overlap slightly. Carefully smooth the dough along the seam with your fingers to secure it. Fold the two short ends of the dough over just to seal the sides, trimming with a sharp knife if they are too long. Smooth the dough at the seams again. Using a pastry brush, brush the egg over the top of the dough, particularly at the seams and cut 3 slits in the top of the dough. Transfer the parcel onto the baking tray.

4   Bake 25 to 30 minutes until the pastry is golden brown, then serve.

Soy cheese is a brilliant dairy-free alternative. Here it provides protein and nutrients, but also a rich taste and a great texture for the covering layer.

Eggplant Parmigiana

Serves **4**   Preparation time **15 minutes, plus making the sauce**   Cooking time **1 hour**

4 eggplants, cut into thick rounds

2 tablespoons olive oil

1½ recipe quantities Roasted Tomato and
    Pepper Sauce (see page 12)

1 small handful of thyme leaves

2 handfuls of basil leaves, chopped

2 cups grated soy cheese

1   Preheat the oven to 350°F. Put the eggplant slices on baking trays and drizzle with the olive oil. Bake 30 minutes, or until golden brown.

2   Add the thyme and a small handful of the basil to the Roasted Tomato and Pepper Sauce and mix well.

3   Put a layer of the eggplant slices on the bottom of a baking dish and cover with one-quarter of the tomato sauce. Sprinkle with a handful of the soy cheese, followed by one-quarter of the remaining basil. Repeat the layers three times, making sure the soy cheese is sprinkled evenly each time, especially on the top.

4   Bake 30 minutes, or until golden brown on top, then serve.

dinners

Lemon thyme has an earthy, aromatic, citrus flavor that works well with the sweet taste of the roasted red onions in this tart.

Roasted Onion, Fig and Lemon Thyme Tart

Serves **4**   Preparation time **15 minutes, plus making the dough**   Cooking time **1 hour 20 minutes**

dairy-free margarine, for greasing

2 red onions, each cut into 8 pieces

2 tablespoons olive oil

brown rice flour, for dusting

1 recipe quantity Light Pastry Dough
  (see page 18), using sweet potato, instead
  of ordinary white potato

4 to 5 figs, stemmed and quartered

2¾ ounces firm tofu or soy cheese

2 extra-large eggs, plus 5 extra-large egg yolks

6 tablespoons unsweetened soy milk

1 large handful of lemon thyme leaves, chopped

sea salt and freshly ground black pepper

1   Preheat the oven to 350°F and grease a loose-bottomed 8-inch tart pan with dairy-free margarine. Arrange the onions on a baking tray and drizzle with the oil. Bake 20 to 25 minutes until starting to brown.

2   Liberally dust a cutting board with rice flour and roll out the dough into a circle slightly larger than the tart pan, to allow enough dough for the side. Be careful as the dough will still be slightly sticky. Neaten the edge with a sharp knife, then ease the dough into the pan, pressing down carefully to remove any air pockets. If the dough looks too fragile to lift into the pan, simply put the pan face-down on top of the dough and turn the board over to drop the dough into it. Neaten the edge again, prick the bottom all over with a fork, then line the tart shell with parchment paper and cover with baking beans. Bake 8 to 10 minutes until just golden. Remove the tart shell from the oven and remove the parchment and beans, then bake 2 minutes longer.

3   Spread the onions and figs over the tart shell, then crumble the tofu or soy cheese over the top. Whisk the eggs, egg yolks, and soy milk together in a bowl, then mix in the lemon thyme and season lightly with salt and pepper. Pour the mixture over the onion, figs and tofu.

4   Bake 30 to 35 minutes until the filling is cooked through. Remove the tart from the oven and let cool in the pan 5 minutes. Carefully ease the tart out onto a serving plate and serve.

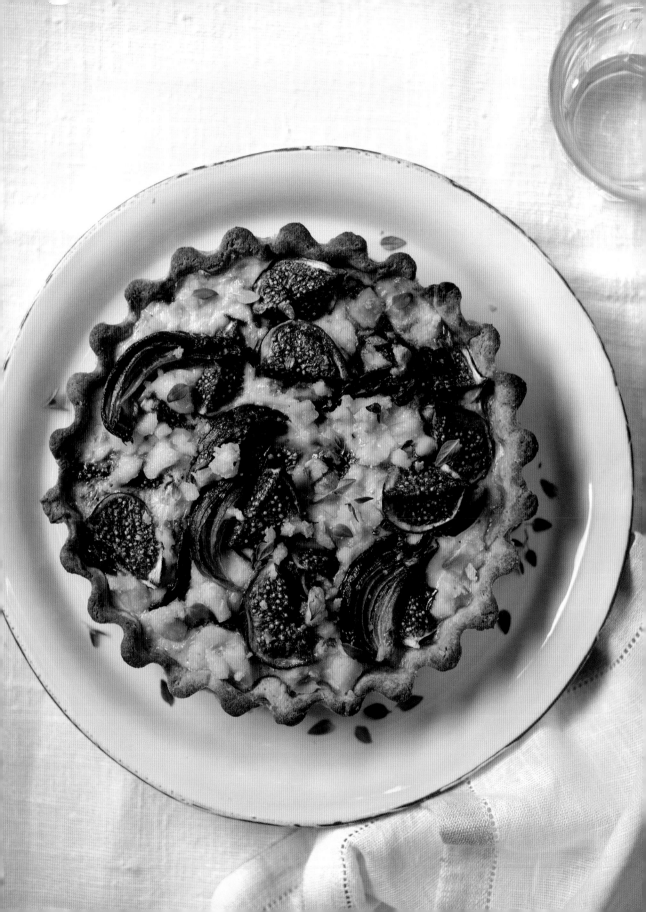

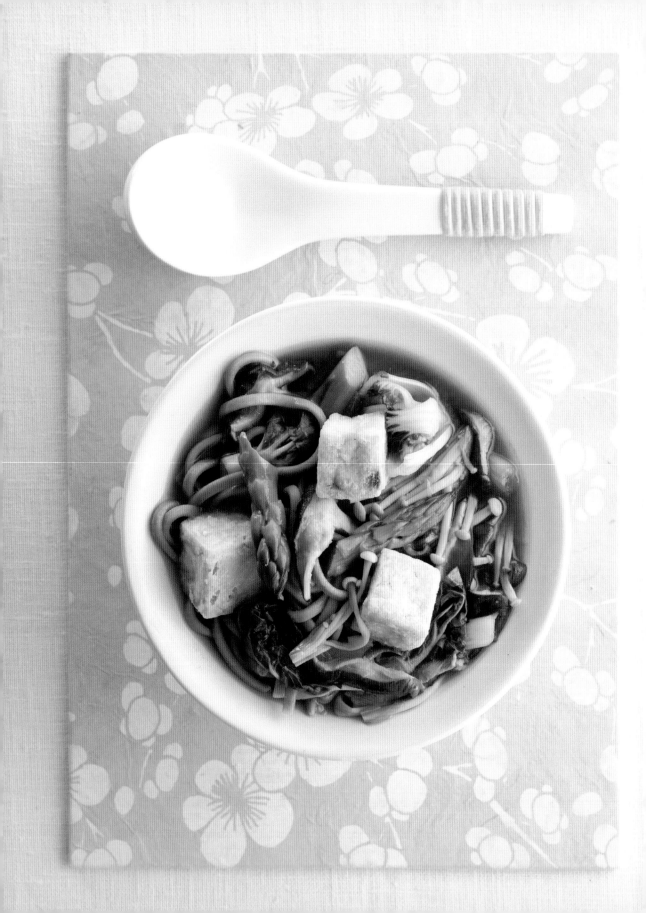

A power-house of nutrients, packed with vitamins, minerals, protein, and essential fatty acids, this recipe uses a gluten-free version of soba noodles, and miso paste and cornstarch to thicken the sauce.

Buckwheat Soba Noodles with Tofu and Miso

Serves **4**   Preparation time **15 minutes**   Cooking time **25 minutes**

1 sheet of kombu

6 scallions, white part only, finely sliced

1-inch piece of ginger root, peeled and finely chopped

2 tablespoons tamari soy sauce

2 tablespoons miso paste

10 ounces mixed Asian mushrooms, such as maitake and shiitake, sliced

2 bok choy, sliced widthwise into thirds, stems and leaves separated

12 ounces asparagus, woody ends discarded and stalks chopped

9 ounces dried 100% buckwheat soba noodles

9 ounces firm tofu, patted dry with paper towels and cut into bite-size cubes

heaped ⅓ cup cornstarch

¼ cup olive oil

1   Put the kombu, scallions, ginger, and 4½ cups water in a large heavy-bottomed saucepan. Cover with a lid and bring to a boil over high heat, then reduce the heat to medium and simmer 5 minutes.

2   Stir in the tamari and miso and then gently stir in the mushrooms, bok choy stems, asparagus, and noodles, making sure the noodles are covered in the liquid. Cover and bring to a boil again over high heat, then reduce the heat to medium and simmer 8 minutes, stirring occasionally to make sure the noodles don't stick together. Add the bok choy leaves and cook 2 to 3 minutes longer until the noodles are cooked, the vegetables are tender, and some broth is still left in the pan. Remove and discard the kombu.

3   Meanwhile, roll the tofu in the cornstarch to coat evenly. Heat the oil in a large skillet or wok over a medium-high heat and add the tofu. Fry, turning occasionally, 5 to 8 minutes until golden. Serve on top of the noodles, vegetables, and broth.

Like all stews, the flavor of a tagine is enhanced when made in advance and then reheated. Store this in the refrigerator overnight or in the freezer for a couple of months for an easy and convenient meal.

Vegetable Tagine

Serves **4**   Preparation time **15 minutes, plus at least 12 hours soaking (optional) and making the stock**   Cooking time **2 hours 15 minutes**

1 cup dried chickpeas or 2 cups drained canned
    chickpeas, rinsed
2 tablespoons olive oil
2 onions, finely chopped
2 garlic cloves, crushed
1 teaspoon cinnamon
1 teaspoon ground cumin
1 teaspoon ground coriander
1½ tablespoons harissa
1 eggplant, chopped into large cubes

3 carrots, cut into batons
1 small butternut squash, peeled, chopped,
    and seeded
½ cup unsulfured dried apricots, chopped
1 cup plus 2 tablespoons Vegetable Stock
    (see page 21) or vegetable stock made from
    gluten- and dairy-free bouillon powder
1 cup slivered almonds
1 handful of flat-leaf parsley leaves, chopped
sea salt and freshly ground black pepper

1   If using dried chickpeas, put them in a bowl, cover with cold water, and soak overnight, or at least 12 hours, then drain and rinse well. Transfer to a large saucepan, cover with fresh water, and bring to a boil over high heat. Boil 10 minutes, then turn the heat down to low and simmer gently, covered, 1 to 1½ hours until tender. Drain well and set aside.

2   Heat the oil in a large, heavy-bottomed saucepan over medium heat. Add the onions and cook, stirring occasionally, 2 to 3 minutes until just starting to turn golden, then add the garlic and cook, stirring, 30 seconds longer. Mix in the spices and harissa.

3   Add the eggplant and cook, stirring occasionally, 5 minutes, then add the carrots and butternut squash and cook 5 minutes longer, still stirring. Add the apricots and stock, turn the heat down to low, and simmer, covered, 20 minutes, or until the vegetables are tender, stirring occasionally.

4   Meanwhile, heat a heavy-bottomed skillet over medium heat. Add the almonds and cook, stirring continuously, 2 to 3 minutes until just beginning to brown.

5   Add the cooked chickpeas and parsley to the tagine and stir well. Sprinkle with the almonds and serve.

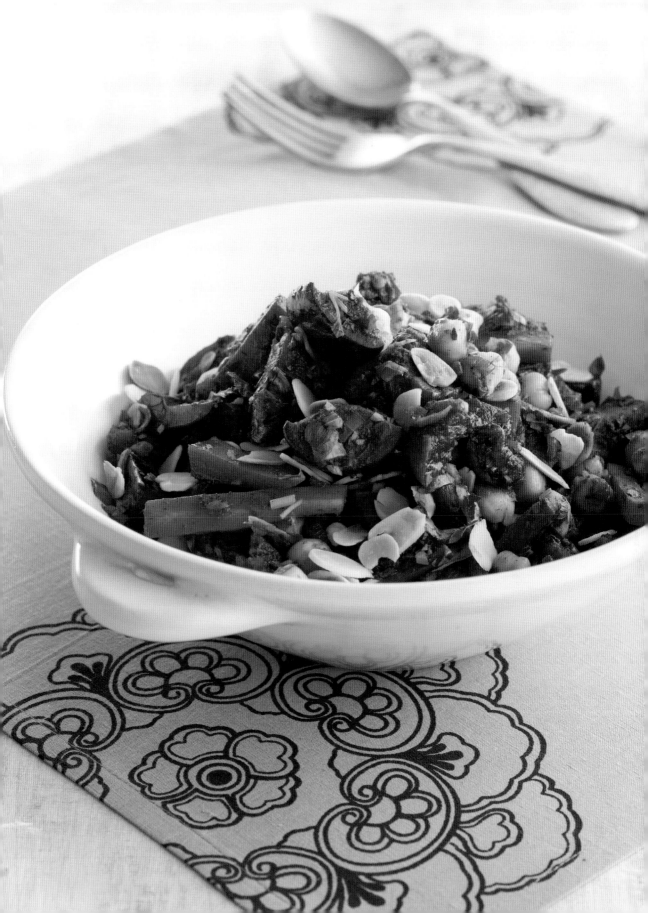

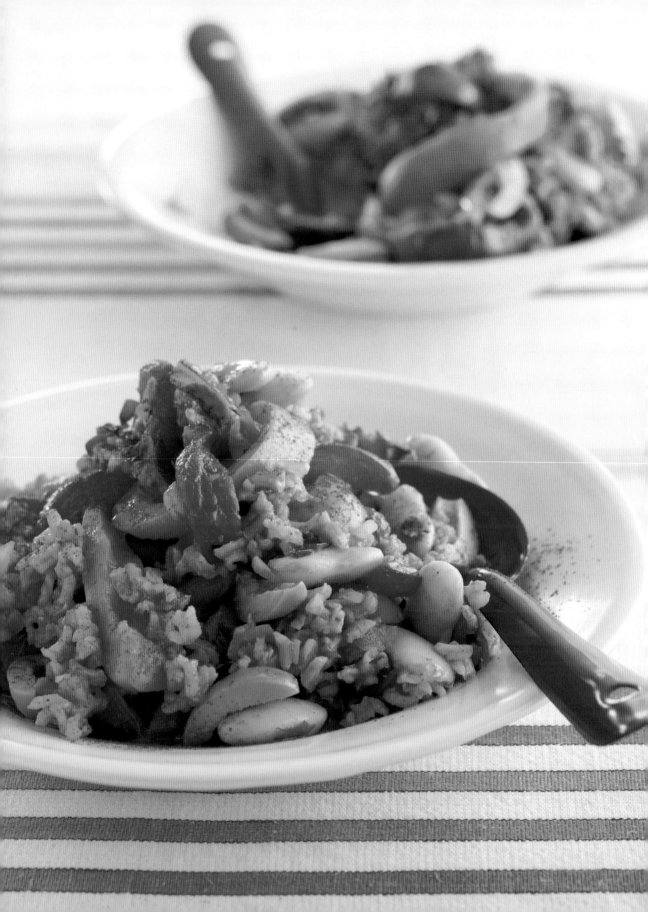

Great Northern beans are my favorite of all the beans. Packed with protein, fiber, and low-GI carbohydrates, they have a firm texture and gorgeous, subtle taste that combines well with strong flavors.

Spanish-Style Beans and Rice

Serves **4**   Preparation time **20 minutes, plus 12 hours soaking (optional) and making the stock**
Cooking time **2 hours 15 minutes**

1½ cups dried Great Northern beans or
  3 cups drained canned Great Northern
  beans, rinsed
6 tablespoons olive oil
1 onion, finely chopped
2 garlic cloves, crushed
1½ tablespoons smoked paprika, plus extra
  to serve
1 tablespoon tomato paste
1½ cups brown basmati rice
1½ cups dry white wine

2½ cups hot Vegetable Stock (see page 21),
  or vegetable stock made from gluten- and
  dairy-free bouillon powder, plus extra if
  needed
6 tomatoes, halved
4 red bell peppers, quartered and seeded
4 orange bell peppers, quartered and seeded
½ cup pitted Spanish olives, chopped
1 large handful of flat-leaf parsley leaves,
  chopped

1   If using dried beans, put them in a bowl, cover with cold water, and soak overnight, or for at least 12 hours, then drain and rinse well. Transfer to a large saucepan, cover with fresh water, and bring to a boil over high heat. Boil 10 minutes, then turn the heat down to low and simmer gently, covered, 1 to 1½ hours until tender. Drain well and set aside.

2   Heat 2 tablespoons of the oil in a large, heavy-bottomed saucepan over medium heat. Add the onion and cook, stirring occasionally, 2 to 3 minutes until just starting to turn golden. Stir in the garlic and cook about 30 seconds, then stir in the paprika, tomato paste, and rice.

3   Add the wine and stock to the pan, cover, and bring to a boil over high heat. Reduce the heat to medium and simmer 35 to 40 minutes until the rice is soft but still has a slight bite and all the liquid is absorbed. Add more stock during cooking, if necessary.

4   Meanwhile, preheat the oven to 350°F. Put the tomatoes and peppers on baking trays and drizzle the remaining oil over them. Roast 25 minutes until tender, then put the peppers in a bowl, cover with a plate, and let stand 5 minutes. Peel off the pepper skins and cut the flesh into chunks.

5   When the rice is almost cooked, stir in the peppers, tomatoes, beans, and olives. When completely cooked, stir in the parsley. Sprinkle with paprika and serve.

Desserts

If you long to eat tarts or pies, cheesecake or creamy ice cream, look no further! Here you'll find mouthwatering desserts ranging from Passion Fruit Curd Tartlets and Cherry Pie, to Blueberry and Lime Cheesecake and Chocolate Semifreddo. But while some of the desserts, like the Chocolate Fondant, are just pure indulgence, many of these recipes are healthy as well as delicious. Dive into Chocolate and Banana Soufflé, for example, instead of the classic chocolate version, Apple and Berry Crumble, or Summer Pudding, both packed with fruit, or Strawberry Pannacotta, made with nutrient-rich cashew nut cream. As my father used to say, it's a sad heart that never rejoices!

Blueberry and Lime Cheesecake, page 158

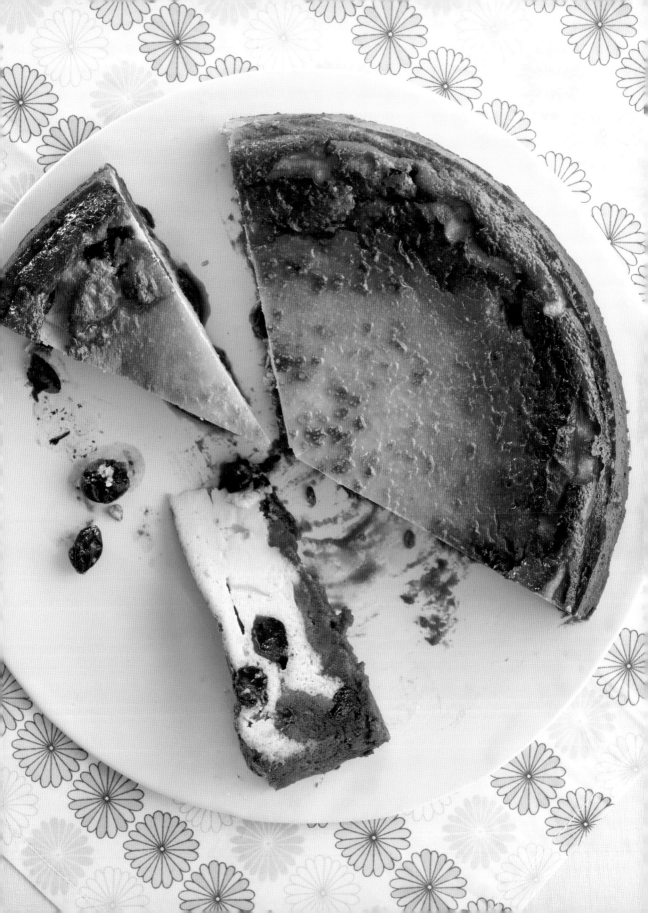

Gluten-free pastry tends to darken and burn very easily. This recipe needs longer in the oven than most tarts, so it's important to check on it toward the end of its baking time and cover it with baking parchment.

Pear and Almond Frangipane Tart

Serves **6 to 8**   Preparation time **20 minutes, plus making the dough**   Cooking time **55 minutes**

5 tablespoons dairy-free margarine, plus extra
    for greasing
brown rice flour, for dusting
1 recipe quantity Sweet Piecrust Dough
    (see page 19)
¼ cup fruit sugar or granulated sugar

2 large eggs
1 cup very finely ground blanched almonds
2 pears, peeled, quartered, and cored
3 tablespoons pear and apricot spread
    or apricot jam

1   Preheat the oven to 350°F. Grease a loose-bottomed 8-inch tart pan with dairy-free margarine and line the bottom with baking parchment. Liberally dust a cutting board with rice flour and roll out the dough into a circle slightly larger than the tart pan, to allow enough dough for the side, then neaten the edge, using a sharp knife. Be careful as the dough will still be slightly sticky. Put the pan, face-down, on top of the dough and turn the board over to drop the dough into the pan. Ease the dough into place, pressing down carefully to remove any air pockets, then prick the bottom all over with a fork. Line the tart case with a piece of baking parchment and cover with baking beans.

2   Bake 8 minutes until just starting to turn golden. Remove from the oven and remove the parchment and beans.

3   Meanwhile, make the filling. Put the dairy-free margarine and sugar in a large mixing bowl and beat, using an electric mixer, until light and fluffy. Gradually beat in the eggs, one at a time, then add the ground almonds and fold together with a spoon until well mixed.

4   Slice each pear quarter into 4 thin slices. Brush 2 tablespoons of the fruit spread over the bottom of the tart shell with a pastry brush, pour in the filling, and cover with the pear slices. Cover the pan with baking parchment, making sure the ends are tucked under the pan.

5   Bake 30 minutes, then remove the baking parchment. Gently brush the remaining tablespoon of the fruit spread onto the pears with a pastry brush and bake 10 to 15 minutes longer until the filling is set. Remove from the oven and let cool in the pan 5 minutes, then carefully ease it out onto a plate and serve.

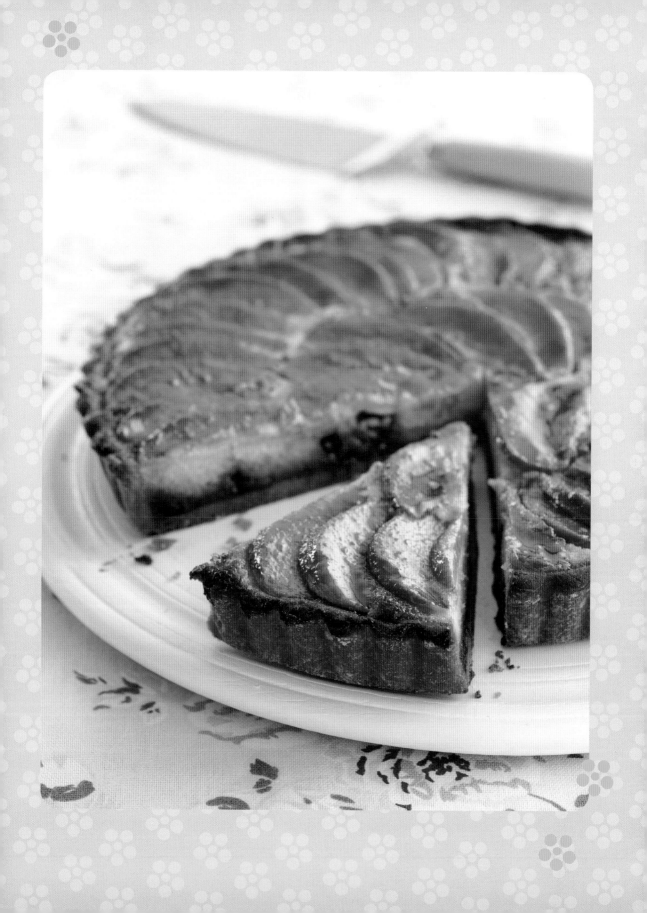

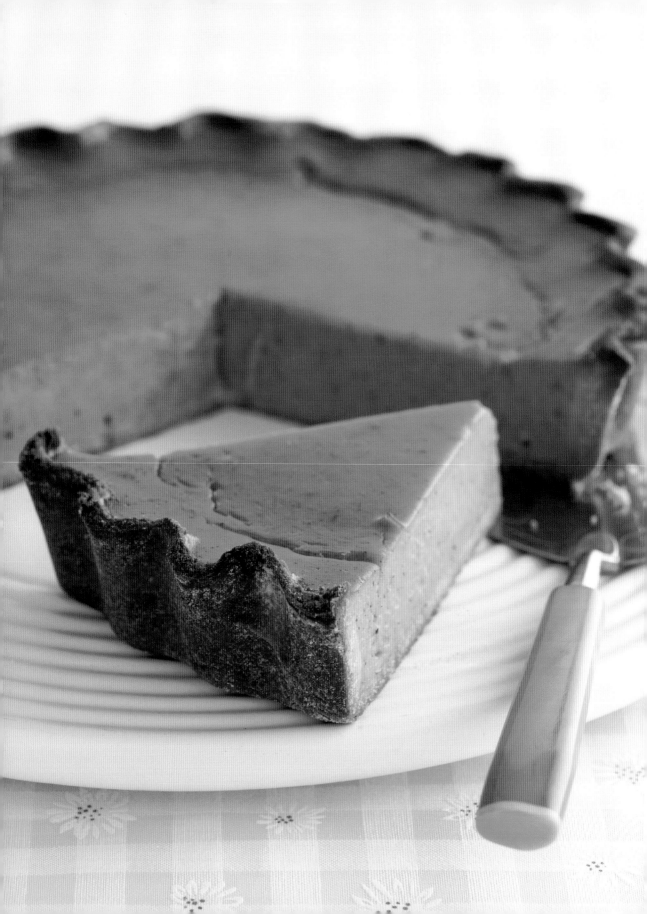

The soy cream works well with the spices, pumpkin, and eggs, making a delightfully rich, creamy pie.

Pumpkin Pie

Serves **6 to 8**   Preparation time **25 minutes, plus making the dough**
Cooking time **1 hour 30 minutes**

3 pounds 5 ounces pumpkin, sliced into 16
    wedges, seeded and fibers removed
dairy-free margarine, for greasing
brown rice flour, for dusting
1 recipe quantity Sweet Piecrust Dough
    (see page 19)

½ cup less 1 tablespoon fruit sugar or
    granulated sugar
1 teaspoon cinnamon
½ teaspoon freshly ground nutmeg
¼ cup soy cream
2 extra-large eggs

1   Preheat the oven to 350°F. Put the pumpkin on a baking sheet, skin-side down, and bake 40 minutes, or until cooked through. Remove from the oven and let cool 5 minutes, or until cool enough to handle, then scoop the flesh into a food processor and discard the skins.

2   Grease a loose-bottomed 8-inch tart pan with dairy-free margarine and line the bottom with baking parchment. Liberally dust a cutting board with rice flour and roll out the dough into a circle slightly larger than the tart pan, to allow enough dough for the side, and neaten the edge, using a sharp knife. Be careful as the dough will still be slightly sticky. Put the pan, face-down, on top of the dough, then, holding the board and pan together, turn them over to drop the dough into the pan. Ease the dough into place, pressing down carefully to remove any air pockets, then prick the bottom all over with a fork. Line the pie shell with a piece of baking parchment and cover with baking beans.

3   Bake 8 to 10 minutes until just starting to turn golden. Remove the parchment and beans and bake 2 minutes longer. Remove from the oven.

4   Meanwhile, blend the pumpkin flesh 5 minutes, or until pureed. Add the sugar, cinnamon, nutmeg, and soy cream and blend well, then add the eggs and blend until well mixed. Pour the filling into the pie shell. Bake 10 minutes, then cover with a piece of baking parchment to help prevent the pastry turning too brown. Bake 20 to 25 minutes longer until the filling is just set but still a little wobbly. Remove the pie from the oven and let cool in the pan 5 minutes, then ease it out onto a plate and serve.

I find gluten-free pastry needs to contain more moisture than the normal kind, making it sticky and hard to handle. But if you use a cutting board and work quickly, you can even make a fully-encased pie like this one.

Cherry Pie

Serves **8 to 10**   Preparation time **25 minutes, plus making the dough and nut cream**
Cooking time **1 hour**

dairy-free margarine, for greasing

2 pounds 4 ounces cherries, pitted

½ cup fruit sugar or granulated sugar

1 tablespoon lemon juice

2 tablespoons cornstarch

brown rice flour, for dusting

1½ recipe quantities Sweet Piecrust Dough
(see page 19)

1 large egg or egg yolk, beaten

½ recipe quantity Cashew Nut Cream
(see page 13) or soy cream (optional),
to serve

1   Preheat the oven to 350°F and grease a 9-inch pie plate with dairy-free margarine. Put the cherries, fruit sugar, and lemon juice in a heavy-bottomed saucepan and heat over low heat, stirring occasionally, 20 to 25 minutes until the cherries are soft. Put the cornstarch and 2 tablespoons water in a small bowl and stir until smooth. Stir the cornstarch mixture into the cherries and cook 3 to 4 minutes longer until the cherry juice thickens.

2   Liberally dust a cutting board with rice flour and set aside one-third of the dough. Roll out the remaining two-thirds of the dough into a circle slightly larger than the pie plate, to allow enough dough for the side, and neaten the edge, using a sharp knife. Be careful as the dough will still be slightly sticky. Put the pie plate, face-down, on top of the dough, then, holding the board and pie plate together, turn them over to drop the dough into the dish. Ease the dough into place, pressing down carefully to remove any air pockets. Neaten the edge, using a sharp knife, then pour the cherry filling into the pie shell.

3   Dust the cutting board again with rice flour and roll out the remaining dough into a circle very slightly larger than the pie plate, to allow enough dough to press down at the edge. Using a pastry brush, brush the rim of the dough already in the pie plate with water. Using a spatula, ease the dough onto the top of the pie and press down around the rim with your fingers to seal and crimp the edge. Brush the top with the beaten egg, then, using a sharp knife, cut a small cross in the middle of the lid to let the steam out during baking.

4   Bake 30 minutes, or until the pastry is a rich golden brown. Leave the pie to cool 5 minutes, then serve hot, drizzled with cashew nut cream, if desired.

desserts

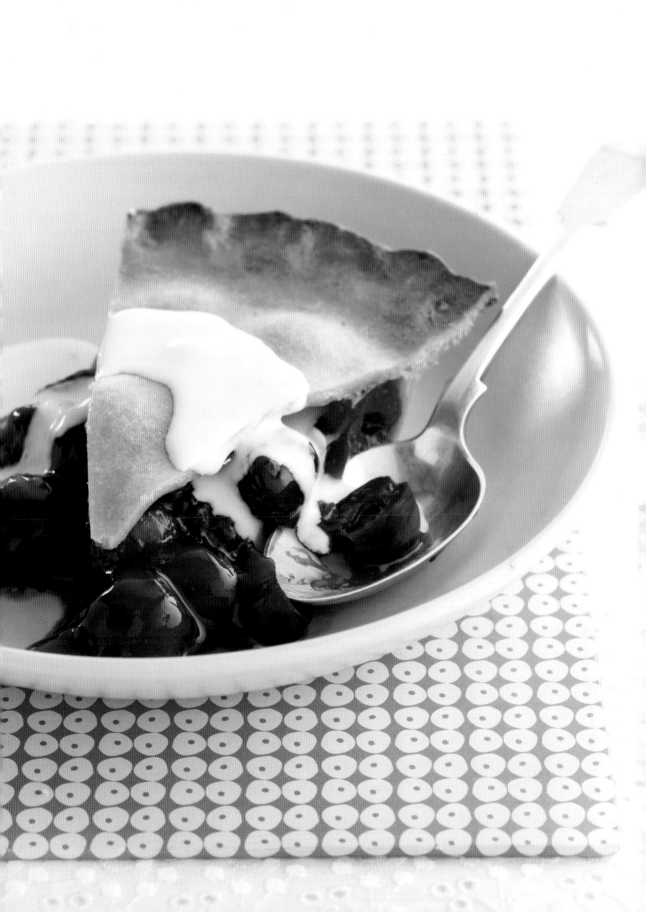

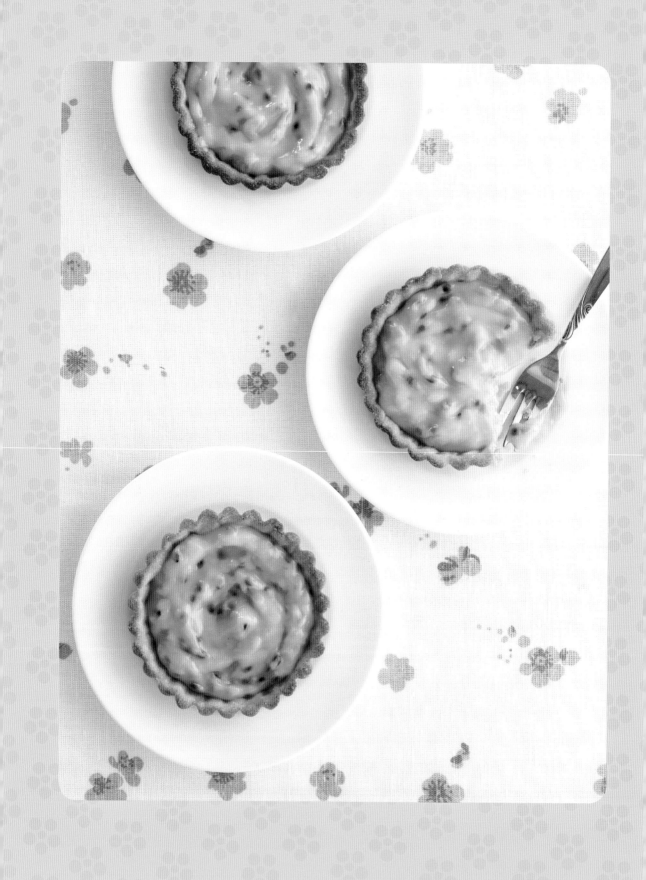

When I was growing up, I adored the lemon curd my mother used to make. This passion fruit version, inspired by her original recipe, has a wonderfully sharp, strong flavor for these tarts.

Passion Fruit Curd Tartlets

Serves **4**   Preparation time **15 minutes, plus making the dough and 30 minutes cooling**
Cooking time **10 minutes**

6 tablespoons plus 2 teaspoons dairy-free
   margarine, plus extra for greasing
brown rice flour, for dusting
1 recipe quantity Sweet Piecrust Dough
   (see page 19)

½ cup less 4 teaspoons fruit sugar or
   granulated sugar
6 passion fruits, halved
1 extra-large egg, plus 3 extra-large egg yolks,
   beaten
1 tablespoon apricot jam

1   Preheat the oven to 400°F and grease four 4-inch tartlet pans with dairy-free margarine. Liberally dust a cutting board with rice flour and gently roll out the dough to about ⅛ inch thick. Using a cookie cutter that is slightly larger in diameter than the tartlet pans to allow enough pastry for the side, cut out 4 dough circles, putting any extra dough in the freezer for use another time. Be very gentle, as the dough will still be slightly sticky. Lift the dough circles into each tartlet pan (you might need to use a spatula) and press down gently to remove any air pockets. Neaten the edges, using a sharp knife, then line each tartlet case with baking parchment and cover with baking beans. Put the pans on a baking sheet and bake 10 minutes, or until firm and light golden.

2   Meanwhile, put the dairy-free margarine and sugar in a large heatproof bowl and rest it over a pan of gently simmering water, making sure the bottom of the bowl does not touch the water. Heat, stirring occasionally, until the dairy-free margarine melts, then scoop the passion fruit seeds into the mixture and add the eggs. Stir until the mixture thickens, then set aside to cool. (If you're not planning to serve the tartlets straightaway, store the curd in the refrigerator once it is cooled.)

3   Remove the tartlet shells from the oven and remove the parchment and beans. Leave the tartlet shells to cool about 3 minutes, then them turn out onto a wire rack and leave to cool completely.

4   Spoon the curd into the tartlet shells and serve immediately. Keep any leftover tarts in the refrigerator up to 1 day.

desserts

These wonderful cheesecakes, filled with sweet blueberries and accented by zesty lime, rich soy cream cheese, and spicy ginger cookies, are a real treat.

Blueberry and Lime Cheesecake

Serves **4**   Preparation time **25 minutes, plus making the cookies and at least 3 hours setting**
Cooking time **40 minutes**

6 tablespoons plus 2 teaspoons dairy-free
    margarine, melted, plus extra for greasing
1 recipe quantity Ginger Cookies (see page 83),
    broken into pieces
2 cups blueberries

scant 2½ cups soy cream cheese
heaped ¾ cup fruit sugar or granulated sugar
zest and juice of 2 limes
4 large eggs

1   Preheat the oven to 350°F. Lightly grease a deep 8-inch springform cake pan with dairy-free margarine and line the bottom with baking parchment. Heat the dairy-free margarine in a saucepan over low heat until it melts. Put the cookies in a food processor and blend until the mixture resembles fine bread crumbs. Add the crumbs to the melted margarine and mix well. Using the back of a spoon, press the mixture evenly into the bottom of the cake pan. Cover with the blueberries and let chill in the refrigerator 10 minutes.

2   Meanwhile, blend the soy cream cheese, sugar, and lime zest and juice together in a food processor until smooth. Add the eggs and blend until smooth and creamy.

3   Pour the cheese mixture over the blueberries and bake 30 to 35 minutes until pale golden brown and the top feels firm to the touch. Turn off the oven and leave the cheesecake to rest in the oven another 30 minutes.

4   Ease the cheesecake out of the pan and let cool completely, then chill in the refrigerator 3 to 4 hours until completely set before serving.

desserts

This is a great recipe for dinner with friends. Make the puddings the night before and use small, individual ramekins to create a stunning dessert.

Summer Pudding

Serves **4**   Preparation time **15 minutes, plus making the cake and at least 12 hours resting** Cooking time **5 minutes**

1 pound 10 ounces summer fruit, such as raspberries, strawberries, blueberries, and red currants

½ cup fruit sugar or granulated sugar
1 recipe quantity Almond Cake (see page 95)

1   Put the fruit and sugar in a medium-size saucepan and heat over low heat, stirring occasionally, 5 to 6 minutes until the fruit softens and the sugar dissolves. Take care not to overcook. Remove from the heat and strain, reserving the fruit in one bowl and the liquid in another.

2   Slice the cake vertically into thin slices with a long, sharp knife. Remove the crusts and cut 3 slices to fit the bottoms of four ¾-cup ramekins or pudding molds. Press gently into the ramekins, so the cake covers the bottoms. Press 3 or 4 more slices around the inside of each ramekin, pressing gently against the sides until covered completely.

3   Divide the strained fruit into the ramekins, filling them to the tops, then cover each one with a saucer and put a heavy weight on top. Chill the ramekins in the refrigerator overnight, or at least 12 hours. Reserve any leftover fruit to serve with the puddings.

4   Remove the weight and saucer from each ramekin and cover with an upside-down serving plate. Turn the ramekins over to turn out the puddings. Remove the ramekins and pour the reserved fruit liquid over the puddings, then serve immediately with any extra fruit, if desired.

*This is melt-in-the-mouth delicious! When you take your first spoonful,
you'll find a rich, gooey, chocolately center inside.*

Chocolate Fondant

Serves **4**   Preparation time **20 minutes**   Cooking time **20 minutes**

6 tablespoons plus 2 teaspoons dairy-free
    margarine, plus extra for greasing
7 ounces dairy-free dark chocolate, 70% cocoa
    solids, chopped or broken into pieces

2 large eggs, plus 2 large egg yolks
½ cup fruit sugar or granulated sugar
2 tablespoons rice flour
heaped 2 tablespoons chickpea flour

1   Preheat the oven to 350°F and grease four ¾-cup ramekins or pudding molds with dairy-free
    margarine. Put the chocolate in a heatproof bowl and rest it over a saucepan of gently
    simmering water, making sure the bottom of the bowl does not touch the water. Heat, stirring
    occasionally, until the chocolate melts. Remove from the heat, add the dairy-free margarine,
    and stir until it melts. Let cool 10 minutes.

2   Meanwhile, using an electric mixer, beat the eggs and egg yolks together in a large bowl. Add
    the sugar and beat until thick and creamy. Using a large spoon, carefully fold in the melted
    chocolate mixture. Sift in the flours and fold until well mixed.

3   Divide the mixture into the pudding molds and bake 12 to 15 minutes until risen and firm
    to the touch. Serve immediately.

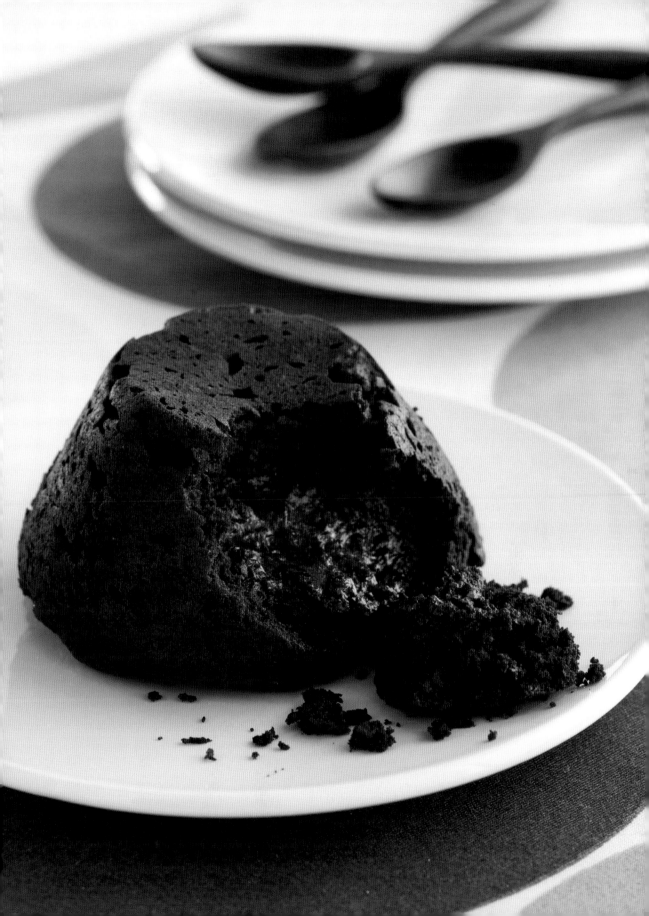

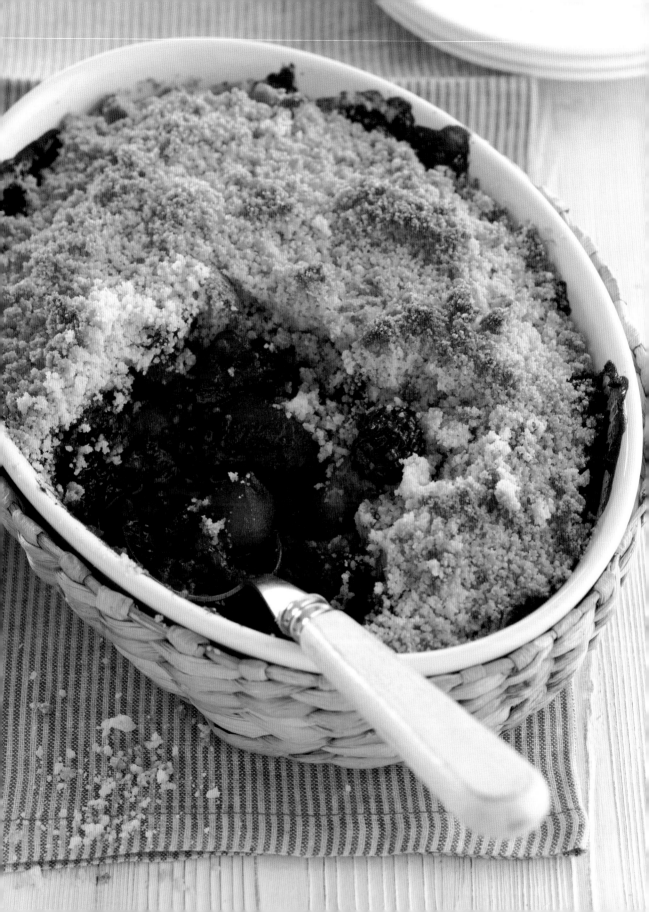

Crumbles are so easy to whip up — and they make a wonderfully wholesome dessert all year around, whether you're using summer or winter fruit.

Apple and Berry Crumble

Serves **4**   Preparation time **15 minutes, plus making the custard**   Cooking time **40 minutes**

3 tablespoons plus 1 teaspoon dairy-free
  margarine

4 apples, peeled, quartered, cored, and cut
  into chunks

2 cups berries, such as blueberries or
  blackberries

3 tablespoons honey

1 recipe quantity Custard (see page 13), to serve
  (optional)

CRUMBLE TOPPING:

scant 1 cup brown rice flour

2 tablespoons corn flour

2 heaped tablespoons chickpea flour

6 tablespoons fruit sugar
  or granulated sugar

6 tablespoons plus 2 teaspoons chilled
  dairy-free margarine, cut into small cubes

1   Preheat the oven to 350°F. Heat the dairy-free margarine in a large, heavy-bottomed saucepan over medium heat until melted. Add the apples and cook, stirring occasionally, 10 minutes, then add the berries and honey. Cook, stirring occasionally, 5 minutes longer.

2   Meanwhile, make the crumble topping. Sift the flours into a food processor, add the sugar, and blend to mix together. Add the dairy-free margarine and blend again until the mixture resembles fine bread crumbs.

3   Spoon the fruit mixture into a baking dish and crumble the topping over, making sure all the fruit is covered.

4   Bake 20 to 25 minutes until browned on top. Remove the crumble from the oven and serve immediately with custard, if desired.

desserts

Here I've used xylitol to make the meringue because fruit sugar doesn't work. The xylitol creates a deliciously squidgy meringue, but if you'd prefer a crunchy, traditional one, simply use granulated sugar.

Eton Mess

Serves **4**   Preparation time **30 minutes, plus making the nut cream**   Cooking time **1 hour 15 minutes**

5⅓ cups strawberries, hulled

5 tablespoons crème de cassis liqueur

3 tablespoons fruit sugar or granulated sugar

½ recipe quantity Cashew Nut Cream
   (see page 13)

MERINGUE:

2 extra-large egg whites

½ cup xylitol or granulated sugar

scant ½ teaspoon vanilla extract

1 Preheat the oven to 275°F and line two baking sheets with baking parchment. To make the meringues, using an electric mixer, beat the egg whites in a large clean bowl until stiff peaks form. Gradually add the xylitol and continue beating until glossy, then beat in the vanilla extract.

2 Spoon the meringue mixture onto the baking sheets to make 6 meringues, spacing them well apart. Bake 1 hour and 15 minutes until lightly golden brown, then remove from the oven and transfer the meringues to a wire rack to cool completely.

3 While the meringues are cooling, cut half of the strawberries into quarters and put them in a large bowl. Add 3 tablespoons of the crème de cassis, toss gently, and let stand 15 minutes.

4 Put the sugar, remaining strawberries, and crème de cassis in a blender and blend well. Strain the mixture through a strainer into a clean bowl to make a coulis.

5 Break the meringues into bite-size pieces and put them in a large bowl. Gently stir the nut cream into the quartered strawberries and liqueur, then fold the mixture into the meringues. Spoon into bowls or glasses, drizzle with the strawberry coulis, and serve.

desserts

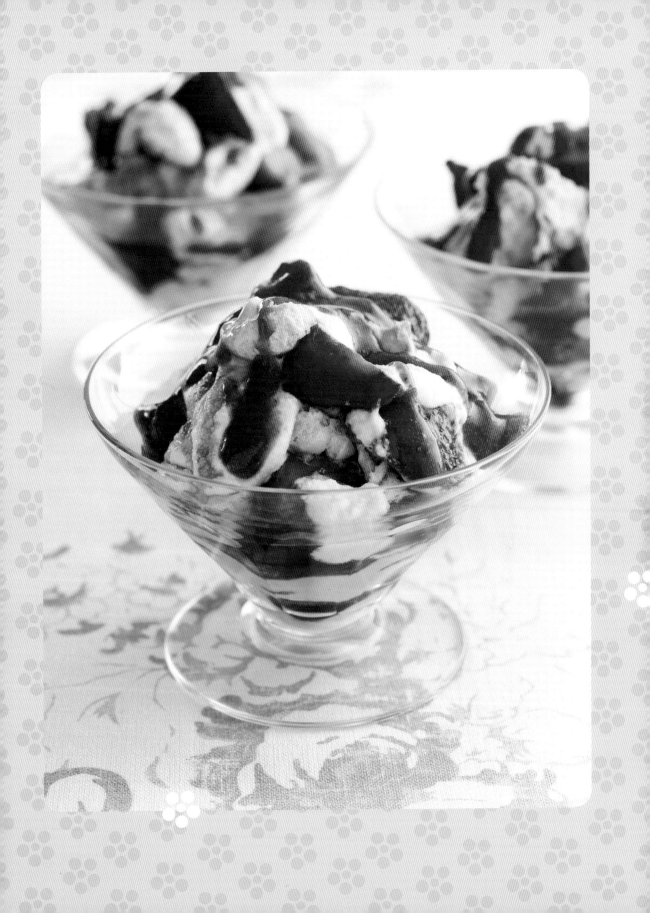

Don't be intimidated by soufflés — they are, in fact, easy to make as long as you whisk the eggs thoroughly and bake at the right temperature.

Chocolate and Banana Soufflé

Serves **4**   Preparation time **15 minutes**   Cooking time **20 minutes**

dairy-free margarine, for greasing

5 extra-large egg whites

½ cup fruit sugar or granulated sugar

3 ounces dairy-free dark chocolate, 70% cocoa
    solids, broken into small pieces

1 tablespoon cornstarch

2 bananas

1   Preheat the oven to 350°F and grease a 2-quart soufflé dish with dairy-free margarine. In a clean bowl, beat the egg whites, using an electric mixer, until stiff peaks form. Gradually add the sugar and continue whisking until glossy.

2   Put the chocolate in a large heatproof bowl and rest it over a pan of gently simmering water, making sure that the bottom of the bowl does not touch the water. Heat, stirring occasionally, until the chocolate melts.

3   Put the cornstarch and 1 tablespoon water in a small bowl and stir until smooth, then whisk it into the chocolate, using an electric mixer, until well blended. Mash the bananas, add them to the chocolate and mix well.

4   Using the washed and dried mixer, whisk one-third of the egg whites into the chocolate mixture until well blended. Then, using a large metal spoon, carefully fold in the remaining egg whites and mix well.

5   Pour the mixture into the soufflé dish and bake 15 minutes, or until very lightly brown on top and well risen. Remove from the oven and serve immediately.

desserts

Pistachios have a great texture and, along with the vanilla, they add specks of color and sweet flavor to this dairy-free custard.

Pistachio Custard Puddings with Roasted Figs

Serves **4**   Preparation time **15 minutes, plus making the nut cream**   Cooking time **40 minutes**

1 recipe quantity Cashew Nut Cream
  (see page 13)
2 vanilla beans, split and seeds scraped out,
  or 2 teaspoon vanilla extract
12 figs or 4 large peaches

3 tablespoons honey
4 extra-large egg yolks
½ cup fruit sugar or granulated sugar
1¼ cups pistachios, shelled
  and finely chopped

1 Preheat the oven to 315°F. Put the nut cream and vanilla beans and seeds, or vanilla extract, in a heavy-bottomed saucepan and heat over low heat 5 minutes, stirring continually to make sure the mixture doesn't burn. Remove the pan from the heat, discard the vanilla beans, and set aside.

2 Put the figs in a baking dish and drizzle the honey over them. Bake 25 to 35 minutes until they are soft, then remove from the oven and set aside.

3 Using an electric mixer, beat together the egg yolks and sugar in a large mixing bowl until thick and pale. Beat in most of the pistachios, reserving a few to use as decoration. Add the nut cream mixture and ¾ cup water and beat until well mixed.

4 Divide the mixture into four 9-ounce ramekins or individual baking dishes and put them in a large baking dish. Add enough boiling water to the dish to reach halfway up the sides of the ramekins. Bake 30 minutes, or, if using vanilla extract instead of vanilla beans, 40 minutes, or until risen, firm to the touch, and starting to turn golden.

5 Sprinkle with the remaining pistachios and serve immediately with the figs.

I've used cashew nut cream here for a thick creaminess and slightly nutty flavor — and agar agar flakes instead of gelatin to set the pannacotta.

Strawberry Pannacotta

Serves **4**   Preparation time **15 minutes, plus making the nut cream and 2 hours chilling**
Cooking time **10 minutes**

2⅔ cups strawberries, hulled

1 tablespoon agave syrup

1 recipe quantity Cashew Nut Cream

   (see page 13)

2 tablespoons fruit sugar or granulated sugar,

   plus extra as needed

1 vanilla bean, split with the seeds scraped out

   and reserved

2 teaspoon agar agar flakes

1   Put the strawberries in a food processor or blender and blend 2 to 3 minutes until smooth. Strain the mixture through a strainer into a clean bowl to make a coulis, then discard the pulp. Put half of the coulis in a measuring jug, add the agave, and mix well. Chill in the refrigerator until ready to use.

2   Put the remaining strawberry coulis in a saucepan and add the nut cream, sugar, and vanilla bean and seeds. Heat over low heat 2 minutes, then taste and add a little more sugar if needed. Sprinkle in the agar agar flakes and cook, stirring continuously, 5 minutes longer, or until the agar agar flakes dissolve. Remove the pan from the heat, discard the vanilla bean, and set aside to cool about 30 minutes.

3   Line four ¾-cup ramekins with plastic wrap. Spoon the cooled pannacotta mixture into the ramekins and smooth the top with the back of a metal spoon. Cover with plastic wrap and let set in the refrigerator at least 1½ hours. Turn out of the ramekins onto plates and remove the plastic wrap. Serve drizzled with the remaining coulis.

desserts

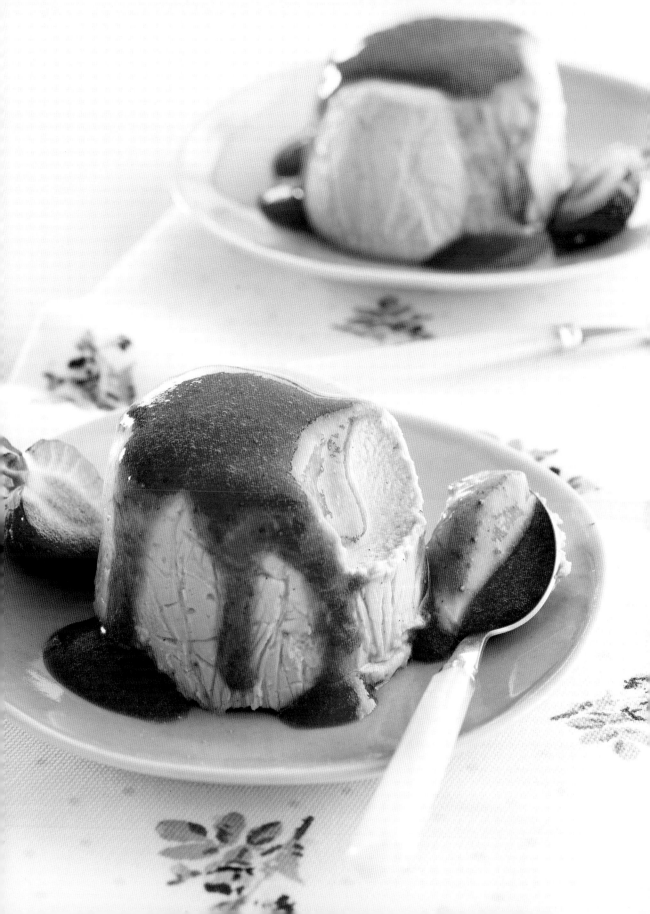

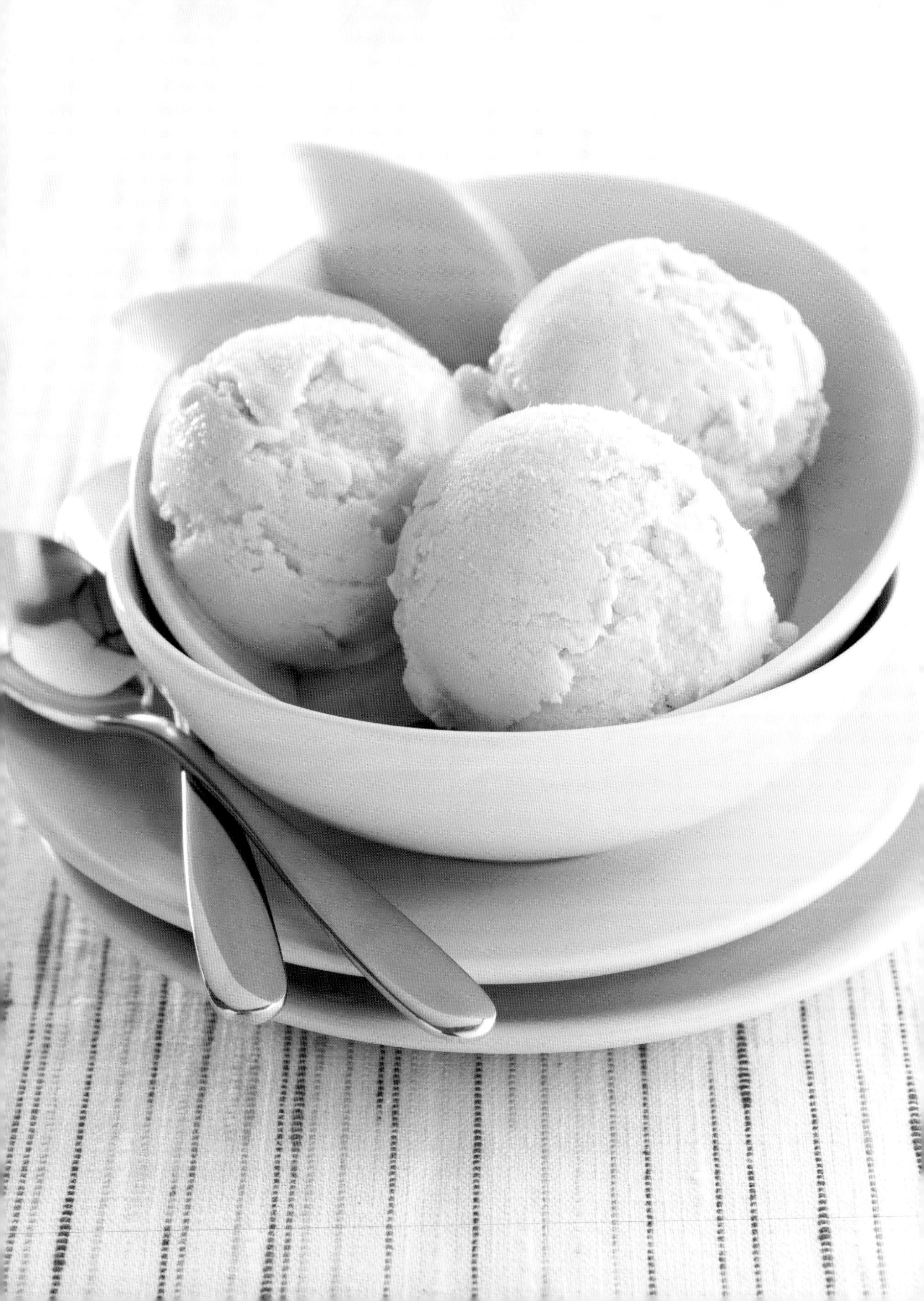

This is a deliciously subtle ice cream, with zesty lemongrass, kaffir lime leaves, and lime juice combining with sweet mango. The key to this recipe is to use beautifully ripe mangoes.

Mango Ice Cream

Serves **4**   Preparation time **25 minutes, plus 8 hours freezing**   Cooking time **5 minutes**

2 cups plus 2 tablespoons soy cream

6 tablespoons fruit sugar
 or granulated sugar

4 lemongrass stalks

25 fresh or dried kaffir lime leaves

1 tablespoon cornstarch

3 very ripe, large mangoes, plus extra sliced
 mango to serve

1   Put the soy cream, sugar, lemongrass, and lime leaves in a medium-size saucepan and heat over low heat until just starting to boil. Simmer 2 minutes, or until the sugar dissolves, stirring frequently. Using a slotted spoon, remove the lemongrass and lime leaves and discard. Put the cornstarch and 1 tablespoon water in a small bowl and stir until smooth. Add it to the soy cream and whisk 2 to 3 minutes until the soy cream thickens a little. Remove from the heat and let cool completely.

2   With a sharp knife, carefully slice each mango down both sides, avoiding the seed. On the inside of each slice, cut the flesh into squares, cutting down to the peel but not piercing it, and scoop out with a spoon. Peel the remains of the mango and slice the flesh from the seed, setting some slices aside for serving. Put the remaining mango flesh in a blender or mini food processor and blend until smooth. Transfer to a large bowl, add the lime juice, and mix well.

3   Using a large spoon, fold the soya cream mixture into the mango. Transfer the mixture to an ice cream maker and process according the manufacturer's instructions.

4   Alternatively, transfer the mixture to a large freezerproof container, cover with a lid, and freeze 2 hours. Whisk the mixture well, using an electric mixer, then return it to the freezer. Freeze 2 hours longer, then whisk again. Freeze another 3 to 4 hours until completely frozen, or overnight.

5   Remove the ice cream from the freezer and let soften slightly 10 to 15 minutes at room temperature, then serve with extra mango slices.

desserts

Whip up this wickedly rich and creamy frozen dessert and enjoy the natural feel-good properties of dark chocolate!

Chocolate Semifreddo

Serves **8 to 10**   Preparation time **20 minutes, plus 30 minutes cooling and at least 3 hours freezing**
Cooking time **15 minutes**

10 ounces dairy-free dark chocolate, 70% cocoa
    solids, chopped or broken into small pieces,
    plus extra chocolate shavings to decorate
scant ½ cup honey

2 teaspoons vanilla extract
2 cups plus 2 tablespoons soy cream
2 tablespoons cornstarch

1 Put the chocolate in a large heatproof bowl and rest it over a pan of gently simmering water, making sure that the bottom of the bowl does not touch the water. Heat, stirring occasionally, until the chocolate melts. Stir in the honey and vanilla extract and mix well, then remove the bowl from the heat and let cool.

2 Meanwhile, put the soy cream in a saucepan and heat over low heat 3 to 4 minutes until just starting to boil. Put the cornstarch and 2 tablespoons water in a small bowl and stir until smooth, then add it to the soy cream and whisk 2 to 3 minutes until the mixture thickens a little. Remove from the heat and pour the mixture into the chocolate. Stir well, then let cool completely.

3 Line an 8½- x 4½-inch loaf pan with a large piece of plastic wrap and pour in the semifreddo mixture. Cover with the plastic wrap and freeze 3 to 3½ hours, or overnight, until set.

4 Before serving, remove the semifreddo from the freezer and let soften slightly at room temperature 10 to 15 minutes. Turn the semifreddo out onto a plate and remove the plastic wrap. Slice and serve sprinkled with shavings of chocolate.

desserts

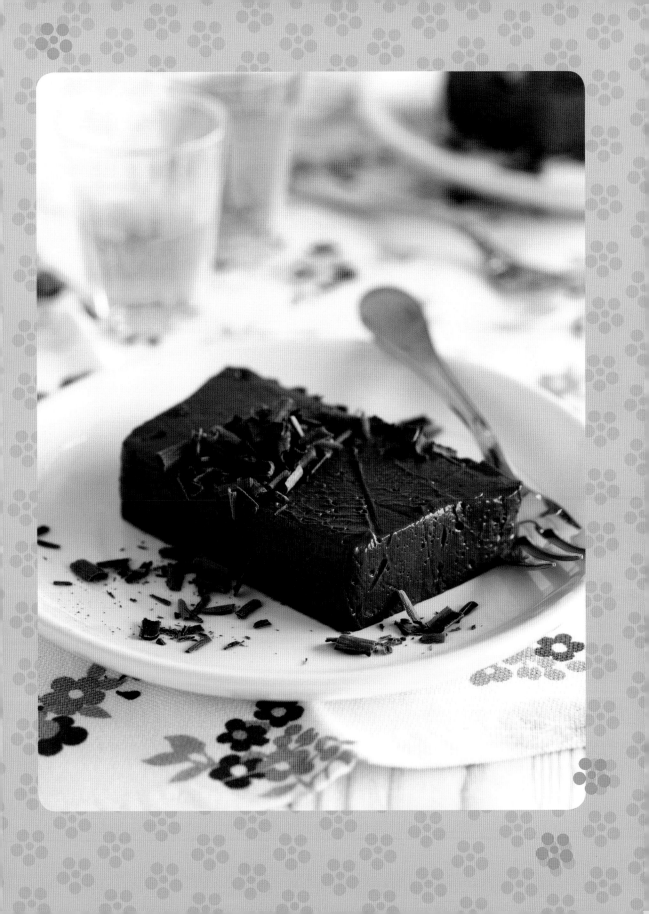

Index

index

index

index